BEYOND the GREY SKY

DUSTIN RUGE

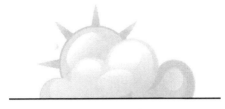

PRAISE

"Dustin Ruge, departing from his previous best-selling books, pours his heart out in "Beyond the Grey Sky." Approaching the 17th anniversary of his brother David's death by suicide, with unvarnished prose and rich anecdotes, he captures the essence of their relationship and his personal journey of healing. Like so many who die by suicide, "David didn't always feel like he 'fit in' to the world we live in." Ruge is a gifted writer – I was transported from laughing out loud (ala David Sedaris) into being moved to tears. This book is a must-read for everyone, not just survivors of suicide loss."

— **Michael F Myers,** MD Professor of Clinical Psychiatry, SUNY Downstate Medical Center, Brooklyn, NY and author of "Touched by Suicide: Hope and Healing After Loss" (with Carla Fine) and "Why Physicians Die by Suicide: Lessons Learned from Their Families and Others Who Cared."

"This is one of the most powerful books on suicide we have ever read. We believe that if everybody could read this incredible story they would not consider suicide. Having known the loss of a loved one to suicide this is one of the most powerful books on suicide we have ever read."

— **Dale and Dar (Darlene) Emme,** Founders of Yellow Ribbon Suicide Prevention Program.

"Beyond the Gray Sky" by Dustin Ruge is his own soul-searching journey in the aftermath of his step brother's suicide. He shares the experience of his shattered world and the Spirit World's subsequent intervention with candor and awe. Ruge's search for meaning in his own life and in his brother's life is compelling. Other suicide loss survivors will relate to his story and will read with curiosity and wonder."

— **Iris Bolton,** Author, Grief Counselor, Director Emeritus of the Link Counseling Center in Atlanta, Georgia. Bolton wrote, "My Son, My Son, A Guide to Healing after Death, Loss or Suicide and recently Bolton Press Atlanta published "Voices of Healing and Hope, Conversations on Grief after Suicide." www.boltonpress.com

"Dustin's story is a heartfelt account about love, grief and our life-long connection we have to our loved ones who have left this world."

— **Friends for Survival, Inc.**

"We, in the field of suicide prevention and support for survivors, have come to understand the value of storytelling to help those in need. Dustin Ruge's story is an excellent example of the power of that storytelling. It is one that should be read by any. I find it invaluable in many situations I have come to work with."

— **Mark Jon Gottschalk,** suicide prevention and survivor support trainer. Member AAS.

"Dustin has written a moving guide for those who have experienced or are experiencing the devastating impact of suicide. In this personal narrative he shares an important perspective of the fraught journey from trauma to acceptance and, eventually, to peace."

— **Dr. Andrew Erlich,** Clinical Psychologist speaker and author of The Long Shadows, www.AndyErlich.com

"Beyond the Grey Sky" *is an honest, painful account that most suicide bereaved will identify with. Ruge gives us permission to explore our relationship with our loved one not just in life, but also in death. Our relationships are necessarily transformed through suicide, but Ruge shows us how the love remains the same and the gifts we can give each other are unchanged."*

— **Melinda Moore, PhD,** Assistant Professor, Department of Psychology, Eastern Kentucky University, Clinical Division Chair of the American Association of Suicidology, and Co-Lead of the National Action Alliance for Suicide Prevention's Faith Community's Task Force."

"Beyond the Grey Sky brings to light the "human factor" and a real look at how suicide impacts not only loved ones, but even acquaintances will be impacted to some degree over such a loss. As a Suicidology Researcher and I know firsthand the tragedy that follows a death by suicide. The "ripple effect" never ceases, the ripples just become less pronounced. However, I know lives can be saved by reading this book."

— **Olivia Johnson, DM,** Blue Wall Institute

"Dustin Ruge has written a book about surviving the loss of his brother to suicide that is personal, engaging and poignant. He gives us a clear picture of the devastation of the death, as well as the strong bond they shared and the growth Dustin experiences after grieving. It is a lovely example of how we can and often do engage with life in a richer way after we work through the heart wrenching aspects of our losses to suicide."

— **Vanessa L. McGann, Ph.D,** Survivors Division Chair, American Association of Suicidology

To my brother David
May you always find your eternal bliss

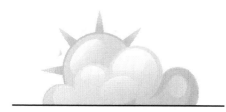

TABLE OF CONTENTS

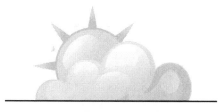

INTRODUCTION

I can't believe you didn't call
What made you want to end it all
Wasn't there something I should have tried
To help you see beyond the gray sky

—311, "Beyond the Gray Sky"

This is a book I never wanted to write and thought I would never finish. As an author of three business books, I have become skilled at writing books in a short amount of time—much to the chagrin of my wife, who has experienced this disappearing act more than once. As an author I also learned that a secret to book writing is to start by drawing a picture of the cover of your new book and placing it over your desk so it is constantly staring down at you, reminding you to finish it. With this book, I created no such book cover, nor did I need to . . . for suicide of a loved one is something that stares you down every day of your life whether you chose it or not.

Many years have passed since I first learned of my brother David's death, but like a picture staring down at me from above, the pain has never really gone away. It has always been there, staring me in my face. Sadly, like many people, I am not alone in this new reality. Just last year I received a call letting me know that one of my first cousins once removed took his own life at the age of twenty-one. Joe Fehr was on a soccer scholarship at Drury University and was an honors student with what seemed like a great life ahead. In his student newspaper he was referred to as "one of the nicest guys I ever met" by friends, and revered by his soccer coach, who said, "I'm at a loss and wish I could have done more." *I know exactly what he means.* Apparently, nobody saw this coming until it was too late. But sadly, Joe's story continues to repeat itself across our nation.

Just the other day I was reading a local Scottsdale newspaper when I noticed an article about two more teens who took their own lives in the East Valley just over the last month. One was a sixteen-year-old valedictorian from Chandler High School and the other was a thirteen-year-old girl. Their deaths brought the total number of teen suicides in this part of the Valley to thirty-five over the past twenty-two months. *Why do I keeping seeing these stories? Why don't people realize how fortunate they really are?*

Having lived through these experiences myself, I never wanted to know much about suicide. To me, it was akin to asking a war veteran about living through the hells of war, which most simply don't want to discuss. I never truly understood why most veterans were this way until my own experiences during the terrorist attacks of 9/11 while living in New York. As a result of that day, I cannot watch images of the planes flying into the Twin Towers or hear recordings of family members talking during their last minutes and seconds with their loved ones before they died. These are moments that bring my own painful memories back into my consciousness, where I never want them to be again. Along with suicide, the painful memories are now seemingly inescapable for me and, sadly, I am not alone.

Approximately one million people worldwide take their own lives each year. In the United States alone, there are around 47,000 suicides per year, and if you are a college student, in the military, part of the LGBTQ community, suffer from autism or mental health or substance abuse issues, you have a higher likelihood of suicide. In my own experience, there were warning signs of suicide in my own family that were either tragically missed, misinterpreted, or, in hindsight, could have been handled differently. *If we only truly knew what could have happened.* In the end it is now the haunting memory of "what could have been if only I had . . . " that is also experienced by so many people who have experienced suicide in their own lives.

Many years have passed since the day suicide first shocked my life and that of my family. As with many things in life, time creates distance, new memories, and new experiences that help us to cover the scars left by suicide. But the scars never really go away; you simply learn to live with them in your world while you assume that those who have carried out suicide have found peace in their own. That is where my story begins and, as you will soon see, how it has changed my view of the world we live in, what suicide really is to me, and the world that lies beyond it.

CHAPTER 1

THE CALL

"Dusty, it's your mother. David is dead. He killed himself."

The day was August 25, 2002, and my wife and I were living in New York and were driving home when I received the call.

"Oh my God!" my wife exclaimed as she broke into tears of disbelief. She seemed to be getting worse with every passing second.

"Calm down, honey," I said after taking a deep breath while trying to keep my cool. This was my standard response to most things in my life after my childhood. I remember years back when my house mother at my fraternity once told my parents upon graduation that I was one of the most "stable" people she had ever met. I never really thought much of her comment at the time, but in situations like this, at least that quality has helped me try to make better decisions under stress.

We were nearly home when we received the call and only a minute later we pulled into the driveway. *Now what the hell do I do?* And where the hell did I miss the instructions on what to do after a family member kills themselves? So, I did what most people would do and started making a rash of phone calls to family members, looking for answers. But here's the problem: When it comes to suicide, there are none. There were only questions that lead to more questions. No answers. David was gone and, at this point, nothing I could say or do would change that fact.

"Mom was the first one to find David," my brother Doug told me over the phone. Since most of us had dispersed from home after growing up, Doug was now my eyes and ears on the ground in Omaha. According to Doug, Mom found David a few days after he took his own life. David's wife, Amy, had left Omaha to attend a close friend's wedding shower in Kansas City and apparently couldn't get a hold of David while she was away. After a few days, she naturally became concerned and my mother drove over to see if there was a problem. I am sure what she saw is a scene from her life she will never forget.

Once David's wife left for Kansas City, David connected a hose from the tailpipe of his truck into the driver's compartment, where he sat. With his car running, the carbon monoxide ended his life then and there. After a few days had passed, the already gruesome scene only got worse and my mother, DEDE, was the first to discover it. I asked her once for more details about that day but I could tell she wasn't comfortable reliving it with me. *Mom was tough but I could tell this was too much even for her.* I am not sure I wanted to know, either—the damage had been done. David was dead and that could not be changed.

This was the first time I had experienced suicide in my life. Like most people, I had heard stories and facts but never really thought it would happen to my immediate family. These are the types of tragedies that only happen to other people, right? That's what I had thought but, as I would soon come to learn, suicide impacts more people than I ever would have guessed.

According to the Centers for Disease Control and Prevention (2017), suicide is the tenth-leading cause of death in the United States with around 47,000 suicides per year, or more than twice the number of homicides. What is more alarming is that suicide is now the second-leading cause of death in people ages ten to thirty-four and second only to unintentional injuries. Put another way, suicide is now the leading cause of "intentional" death amongst America's youth.

To make matters worse, suicide rates have been INCREASING by 30 percent over the past fifteen years alone. Unless these growth trends are reversed, it is very possible that suicide could become the number-one killer of our youth over the next few decades alone. David was thirty-two years old when he died and, as the numbers show us, he was by no means alone. *BUT WHY? WHAT THE HELL IS GOING ON HERE?*

Once the dust had settled, David's body was cremated and laid to rest in an urn next to his biological mother's ashes in the Barker family plot. Besides the funeral I attended after 9/11 in New York *(next chapter)*, it was perhaps the most surreal funeral service I have ever attended in my life.

I have experienced a good deal of tragic death in my life. It all started for me at the age of six when I attended the funeral for my father, Doug Ruge, who died suddenly at the age of thirty-six. Dad died on Father's Day, 1977, of a massive heart attack while returning from a social gathering at a remote location called "the property," about an hour from Omaha.

According to my mother's account of that day, Dad was not feeling well at the party and asked Mom to drive them home. After a short distance, Dad suddenly shot up out of the front seat, landing in the back seat, and told my mom, in apparent excruciating pain, "Take me to Methodist Hospital." Those were his last words to my mother before he passed. When they finally arrived at the emergency room at Methodist Hospital, Mom could overhear one of the medics say to another that he was "already cold." *My poor mother! I can only imagine what that hour in the car must have been like for her.* Sadly, this would not be her last experience as an eyewitness to tragic death.

If you have ever lost your father, especially at a young age, you know what a life-altering event it can become. To lose him on Father's Day was simply adding insult to injury and has turned what should be a time of annual dad-spoiling into a hallow anniversary full of "what ifs" and "could have beens" for my brother and me. Even to this day, I cannot hear "Happy Father's Day" without thinking of my own father first.

By all accounts, our father, Doug, was a remarkable man who was called home at a frightfully young age. My memories of my father are not as vivid as those of my older brother Doug Jr. but there are moments I do recall, albeit through the lens of a six-year-old child. Most of my understanding of my father came from comments and stories of those older than me who knew him best. Dad attended military school, which I am certain helped mold him into the properly kept and highly ambitious person that he was.

Dad was an entrepreneur in the truest sense of the word. At the time of his death, he was active in multiple businesses and ventures along with a monumental effort to save a historic building—the famed Woodmen of the World Building in downtown Omaha—from destruction. At the time of its construction, the Woodmen building was in a class by itself and was the tallest building between Chicago and the West Coast.

For those of you who may be new to Omaha: Yes, we built a historic building full of Italian granite and terracotta architecture that would never be seen again if it were destroyed. Dad clearly understood this, which is why he tried to save it from becoming the casualty of a new city park. But his premature death meant an end to many of the monumental accomplishments and dreams of his short life, including stopping the destruction of this historic building. I still remember sitting at a friend's house that was located close to the building on the day it was demolished. I can still see the dust cloud rising into the sky while the local politicians must have been onsite and smiling in awe. *This was my first major lesson in loathing politicians.*

According to his will, my father wanted to be cremated. My mother decided instead to bury our father so we kids could have somewhere to visit him. Clearly Mom wore the pants in the family! *Thanks, Mom!* Based on the attire they wore back in the mid-1970s I'm sure Dad, if he kept up on fashion trends, now regrets Mom's decision here. Nobody wants to be buried in a 1970s polyester-and-plaid seersucker suit—I sure as hell don't! Oh, well; that's for them to argue over when they meet again. Prior to Dad's burial fashion show, I placed a letter I had written to my father in his casket during the service. Mom had asked me if I wanted to kiss him and I remember saying no. I'm not sure why I made that decision at that time but I'm sure the last thing my mother wanted to do was argue with a confused and angry six-year-old looking for answers to a life tragedy. *Smart move, Mom!* It was a difficult day for everybody and sadly something I would unknowingly experience again twenty-five years later with the death of David.

David's funeral service was held at All Saints Episcopal Church in Omaha. In many respects, All Saints was our "family" church and one that our stepfather, Joe Barker, was an active member of. The Barker family has a long lineage to both Omaha and the Episcopal Church (formerly the Church of England), dating back to the 1860s. During the span of the 1860s to 1871, Joseph Barker, Jr. wrote more than two hundred letters back home to his family in England about his experiences in Omaha. With the great westward expansion and railroad heading west, Omaha had quickly become a thriving and rapidly growing launching point for Americans heading west. These letters are now published in a two-book series entitled *Their Man in Omaha— The Barker Letters (Volume I and II).* If you are an

American history buff, this is a great read about what it was really like in the early American west.

The man who wrote these letters, Joseph Barker, Jr., later became the Right Reverend Joseph Barker, Jr. and once preached in a church in Omaha that my oldest brother, Scott, of the same namesake (Scott was his nickname from his official name of Joseph Scott Barker), would later preach in himself. *Small world, right?* But our stepfather, Joe, although not part of the clergy, was about as close as you could get to it without changing careers.

When our families joined together in 1979, we were introduced weekly to All Saints Church with a loud and bellowing Joe Barker, who sang louder from the pews than the choir did from behind the altar. Let me tell you a little trick I learned from Joe: If you want your kids to quickly escape to Sunday school from service, sing as loudly as you possibly can so you can both embarrass your kids and draw stares from all the people around you. Trust me—it works! But just because religion played a large part in some of our lives didn't mean others, including David, weren't more skeptical.

I'm not exactly sure what David believed in, but having grown up with him, I can confidently tell you that church was not something we both looked forward to and, when we had the option, was not on the Sunday agenda by choice. So how ironic that services for David were now held in one of the places that he would have wanted to be in the least. After the service, we all congregated at the Barker family burial plot, where the urn with David's ashes was placed next to his mother's and then lowered into the ground. David's wife, Amy, then placed a note and picture next to David's remains. At that point, I lost it. It was too many memories and too much déjà vu for me all at once. It was a good thing I had my wife's back to bury my head into and cry. I couldn't keep my cool any longer and had to let it go.

At the time of David's funeral service, I thought this would be the end where, somehow, I would find some semblance of closure and be able to move on. What instead awaited me was a life-altering discovery and awaking that only David's death could bring about and is what led me to share these stories with you. But this was not what my own experiences up to this point in my life had taught me.

After the death of my father and other people in my life up to this point, I had taught myself to accept that "everything happens for a reason" and that the best way to move on is to find closure, accept this time of mourning, and get on with life. But what happened in the months and years that followed David's death not only changed what I believed about suicide and death but are also to this day things I do not fully understand but can only explain from what I experienced. And as I would soon learn, my attempt at a quick "closure" was not an option. Not for me, and apparently not for David.

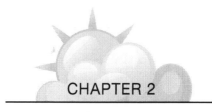

CHAPTER 2

9/11

Our journey to New York certainly wasn't starting out as planned. Only a month after first moving to New York from Atlanta to start our family, we received a call equally as devastating as the one about David. It was September 11, 2001, and I was sitting in my office when I received a call from my wife, Joanie.

"Where are you?!" she nervously shouted over the phone.

"What do you mean?" I responded while sitting in my isolated office getting my workday started. I am not one for office "coffee talk" and other distractions, so when I initially heard some commotion in the lobby of our office, I paid it little mind. This typically works well day to day in the business world when it comes to productivity, but as I soon discovered, today was not that day.

"Haven't you seen the news yet?! The Twin Towers have been hit and we are heading over to Mom's house now!" Joanie yelled over the phone.

"Okay, I'm heading there right now," I replied as I rushed out into the lobby, where a group of people were huddled around a TV watching the live coverage of the World Trade Center towers burning. My father-in-law worked there. *Holy shit!*

I proceeded to drive down the Long Island Expressway at speeds that rivaled my early years as a NASCAR driver. If there was ever a period where time seemed to stand still, that was one of them. Now, I can only imagine what this seemingly endless journey must have been like for my mother twenty-four years earlier with her husband—my father—dying in the back seat of her car. *When the hell will I finally get there?!*

When I finally arrived at my mother-in-law's house, everybody was standing around the TV, which was broadcasting the events as they unfolded. At the time, both towers had been hit and everybody was getting really concerned. Nobody seemed to know what was happening—including the moron TV anchors, one of whom asked on-air how they could get that plane out of the building. *Seriously!? And I thought politicians were the dumbest people on earth. Time to rethink that.*

And then it happened: The first of the two towers collapsed. At that point, I could only hear my in-laws screaming and crying. The air just got sucked out of the room and at that point, we all started to wonder if Charlie was still alive. My father-in-law, Charlie, was working that day in the tower where the second plane hit. Call after call was frantically made to Charlie's mobile phone with no answer. *Was he still alive?* All we could do was wait, and wait. Minutes seemed like hours and then the second building collapsed and still no answer from Charlie's phone. It was starting to look bleak and many in the room were losing hope.

Strangely, while the world was seemingly crashing down around us, I will never forget how beautiful the weather outside was that day. I remember walking out on their back deck and gazing toward the New York City skyline, trying to see a sign of the destruction. All I saw was a beautiful blue sky with calm waters below, standing in stark contrast to the hell that was unfolding beyond it. It was surreal and one of those moments in life that I will never forget. And then, after what seemed like an eternity, we got word: Charlie was safe.

It turned out that the cell phone towers in New York City were overloaded with calls during this time and it was next to impossible to get through to anybody. *Yeah, we kind of figured that out on our own!* Charlie was safe and now we needed to get him home. One of their neighbors, Joe Grassetto, decided to drive to the Brooklyn Bridge to pick

Charlie up and drive him home. Joe was always one of my favorite people in New York and this was yet another reason in my mind why the world needs more people like Joe in it. Now all we could do was wait . . . and watch.

America had not witnessed an attack on its soil like this for over sixty years and the country, and the world, was now in shock. During Pearl Harbor, the Japanese launched a sneak attack by plane while on 9/11, in New York, the terrorists did their own kamikaze show on a grand and sickening scale. But aerial attacks were not the only thing they had in common, for as we would learn in the months and years that followed, both events could have been prevented. There were plenty of warning signs that could have been better interpreted to help prevent these attacks, but in both cases, most people simply didn't or couldn't see them coming until it was too late. As I would learn a year later, suicide can cause you to live with the same regrets.

After waiting hours for his return, Joe finally pulled up with Charlie in the passenger seat. He got out with a handheld radio in one hand and McDonald's in the other. He was quickly surrounded by his emotionally drained and relieved family members. *Wow, were we lucky!* But after listening to Charlie's story about that day, we never knew how close we really came to losing him. It all started when the first tower was hit.

After the first plane hit the North Tower, Charlie could see the damage from the South Tower, where he was working that day. Charlie said he could hear the emergency broadcasting system in the South Tower telling people to remain calm and to not evacuate.

"I knew something was wrong," said Charlie. "I was there during the '93 bombings and this didn't feel like an accident to me."

Charlie then decided that even in bad times, nature still calls, and decided to go to the restroom. While standing over the urinal, the second plane struck about twenty floors above him, knocking him off his feet.

"It felt like the building was going to fall over and I thought that was it," said Charlie. The building swayed back and forth around him. As Charlie later explained to me, the Twin Towers were uniquely designed with an external structural exoskeleton that made the towers literally "sway" in heavy winds. So, when the force of the airliner hit the structure, the towers apparently did what they always did under force, only this time Charlie thought it might be too much. *Once again, another life event that cannot be fully experienced by watching TV alone.* After the building stopped swaying, Charlie proceeded to evacuate down the emergency stairwells.

On his way down, he ran into two frightened girls who were running up to the roof, where they thought they could be safe. Charlie stopped them both and was able to convince one of the two girls to head back down, thereby saving her life. On his way down, Charlie also received a distress call from a stuck elevator. There was nothing he could do to help them and told them to follow the emergency procedures. *I could tell this was the beginning of his survivor's guilt.* Once he reached the ground level of the building, he made his way in the direction of the Brooklyn Bridge while carefully avoiding the falling debris and bodies all around him.

Charlie was one of the many survivors, families, and dignitaries who were invited back to the site of the Twin Towers during the first anniversary of the attack of 9/11. At that time, there was nothing left but a big hole in the ground where the towers once stood, which people now referred to as "Ground Zero." I share this story because even to this day, it still makes the hair stand up on my arm when I hear it. According to Charlie, here is how it went:

Much like the year before, it was a peaceful and calm day in downtown Manhattan. As they stood around the former site of the Twin Towers, a moment of silence was observed at the exact time that the attack took place one year earlier. Charlie then noticed something strange. Out of nowhere came a large gust of wind down the street leading to Ground

Zero. Once the gust hit the site, it swirled up high into the air, filled with dust from the site where the buildings once stood. Charlie said that he knew it was some sort of sign or message. Once he returned home, walked through the front door, and saw his best friend Glenn's name appear on the TV screen while the network played a reel of the 2,996 names who lost their lives on 9/11, he was convinced it had all happened for a reason. *Coincidence?* I don't know for sure, but to Charlie it wasn't.

Once things settled down a bit at the in-laws, we decided to drive home and make sure our dog, Husker, was doing okay. As we drove up our street, something was odd. Why were all these cars parked around our neighbors' house? What happened to the O'Neills? After a while, I finally mustered the courage to walk over and find out for myself. It was not the news I wanted to hear.

The O'Neills' twenty-one-year-old son was working for Cantor Fitzgerald, which was located at the top of the Twin Towers. *Unbelievable!* Here I was telling them about the safe return of Charlie while trying to help them stay confident that their son may have survived. As it turned out with every employee of Cantor Fitzgerald working in the towers that day, he never returned home. I still remember looking at the O'Neills that day in their home and not knowing what more to say to them. That look of stunned and helpless disbelief on their faces was something I still to this day cannot fully describe. Sadly, I would see this look again and far sooner than I ever would have thought.

It was now eleven months after 9/11 when I received the call. My brother David is now dead from suicide. My world just tragically changed again!

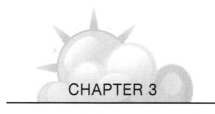

CHAPTER 3

THE BARKER BUNCH

"The world is a comedy to those who think and a tragedy to those who feel."

—Horace Walpole

"I still can't believe we all survived" is what we kids used to joke amongst ourselves when reflecting on our rambunctious and unbridled adolescence. Growing up in a blended family is not easy but somehow, some way, we did it. Notwithstanding any Omaha Police Department cold case files on missing lawn statues, exploding mailboxes, property damage, and the like, we were convinced that we beat the odds and all made it as one blended family.

We were the "Barker Bunch," but nobody who knew us at that time would ever have confused us with the popular TV family the Brady Bunch. Yes, we were a blended family, but that's where the similarities ended. In our new blended family there was no AstroTurf lawn, no family singing groups, and no problems with the sudden zit ruining a prom. In our new world, the lawn was divided to be mowed for money, which was usually spent on beer and other means of escape; the family rarely got together for anything, including "family" dinners; and most of us never left a pre-party to even make it to our own high school proms. Our childhood was so unhinged at times that it was not uncommon in later years for us to gather and joke about how it was amazing we all survived. That is until this day, when all of our worlds were rocked to the core . . . together. The easiest way to picture our family during those times would be to imagine blending *The Brady Bunch* with *Animal House.* Now you can start painting the picture.

It all started back in 1979 when my widowed mother DEDE married the widower Joe Barker III. Both had lost their spouses a few years prior to tragic and unexpected deaths. My father, Doug, died of a massive heart attack brought on by arterial sclerosis while Joe's wife, Susie, died in her sleep. At that point, both DEDE and Joe had to deal with the fallout of their losses in addition to caring for five young children, all of whom were at an age where BB gun wars, partying, and alcohol were firmly taking hold. *Those poor bastards—they didn't have a chance with us!*

Once they met and decided to get married, we began the blending process. I will never forget the day of the wedding when Father Pete, who was the long-standing minister at All Saints Episcopal Church *(Does that place sound familiar yet?)* pulled us kids aside in the waiting room to tell us that the odds of a blended family surviving were not good and it would be up to us to make it work. Let's see; we were five unruly kids with practically no similarities, spanning eight years of age, with a new parent for each side who in many respects was very different than the parent they replaced. *What could possibly go wrong?*

Father Pete was right, though. Blended families, although becoming more common in society today, have terrible success rates. Although the government seems to lack accurate statics on the survival rates of blended families, it is generally accepted that nearly 60–70 percent of blended families with children will not survive. To put this into perspective, that's around twice the failure rate of all marriages. Yet despite the odds, most remarriages today involve children from a previous marriage. *I always knew my stepfather, Joe, liked to gamble, but this had to have been his biggest bet by far.*

As I would soon learn from the "blending" experience, putting a family together is a lot like working with a jigsaw puzzle with a few missing pieces. In some respects, losing a mother or father you were close to in your first family is a piece that simply cannot be replaced either in part or in whole in your new blended family. Even though your new mother or father may now exist, the bonds can be hard to form and accept and, in our own experiences, have sometimes taken many years to truly take hold. I think this has more to do with the kids finally growing beyond the age of "knowing everything" and the parents finally calming down and stop trying to be all things to all people. At least for us, this took a good deal of time, dedication, persistence, and perhaps even luck. *Father Pete knew what he was talking about.*

From the Barker side entered two new brothers and one sister. Scott was the oldest and nearing the end of high school, followed by Amy and then David. On the Ruge side, my brother Doug was nearly three years older than me, while I was now, once again, the youngest child in the family. Yah— think I got any shit for that? David was only one year and one class grade my senior, which means that chronologically we should be the most likely to mesh, which we did. But as we grew and matured, our life paths would take us in very different directions and, in the end, back again. But that would come later. For now, we were both around ten years old, we both lived on our bicycles, loved fireworks and getting in trouble, and we both were dead-eye shots with a BB gun. *The perfect new brother!*

We moved our blended family together to the Ruge home on 90th Street, which is how it was always referred to moving forward. The property was purchased by my parents shortly after I was born and sat on nearly five acres of land located in Omaha's highly desirable District 66 school district. Except for Scott, who wanted to finish out his high-schooling at Central High, we all worked our way through this school system in our respective grades. This was a smart move by the parents, who we now affectionately referred to as "the rentals." *Yes, we were that bad!*

90th Street consisted of a main house and an adjoining but smaller "little house," which was to become as familiar to our friends as it was to the Omaha Police Department. Across the circular driveway was a two-story garage/barn constructed by my father shortly before his death and a backyard tennis court that found more use in the winter months as a neighborhood hockey rink complete with blood-stained ice from the constant checking of hated friends and neighbors into a surrounding sharply spiked corrugated fence. I hear there were some games of tennis played there as well, but I never saw the blood to prove it. *Just kidding . . . sort of.*

The older kids got first dibs on the little house, which meant that Scott and Amy, followed by Amy and Doug, were the benefactors of pre-Animal House living before they moved on to college to "calm down." Parties at the little house were seemingly never-ending and our parents seemed to turn the other way at our rambunctious adolescence antics that took place nightly on the very property they lived on. Despite all this, however, there were times when us kids had to interact with the rentals. This commonly ranged from the occasional car wrecks involving the older kids—sending our family auto insurance premiums into the stratosphere—to the most innocuous driving of David and I to our soccer and football games in wet uniforms that only found their way into the dryer minutes prior to leaving for our games. *Thanks, Mom!*

As we kids started to mature *(in age, that is)*, David and I were largely denied the freedom first afforded to the others, who were fortunate enough to move into the little house, thereby starting their college lifestyles shortly after puberty. Now that we were the last two chickens left in the nest, the rentals decided to rent out the little house, leaving us with no other choice but to contain our debauchery under their own roof. This meant moving into the basement of the main house, where a separate bedroom, bathroom, living room, and a built-in bar were awaiting us and our friends.

I've always wondered what the rentals were thinking by letting all this happen under their own roof. Many people growing up today would gasp at hearing about such an unbridled adolescence, yet back then, it went on largely unabated. Why? This was the question I asked them a few years back and here is how they responded:

"If you and your friends were going to drink, the last thing we wanted was to have you all driving around and putting yourself and others in danger at the same time," is what they told me. I had to let that settle in a bit, but after careful consideration I could fully understand the methods to their madness. After all, we were not out drinking and driving most nights and many of our friends were also the sons and daughters of their own friends, so they were doing us all a favor. Now, I realize some will read this and may strongly disagree with our upbringing, which is fine. I am not writing this to impress or offend you. This is simply how it was and if you take offense to that, well, you are free to go be miserable somewhere else.

Over time and as we matured, all of our lives took starkly different turns and directions. If our lives were a blender, you couldn't have mixed a more contrasting group of ingredients than those our two families provided. If the odds were against us to begin with, then we must have been at the highest risk of any number.

As previously discussed, David and I were the two youngest members of our blended family and seemed to share a lot more in common at the time than in our later years. Once our family "blended," David and I quickly discovered a power play on our parents *(once again, now referred to as the rentals)* that would make any hockey team envious. It was five on two now—what a power play! The rentals now had so many things on their plates while we had a seemingly infinite amount of time, fireworks, and acres of good hunting grounds, plus an unlimited supply of BBs courtesy of the rentals maintaining an open charge account at the countryside hardware store, only a short bike ride from our house. The rentals maintained similar charge accounts at both the clothing store and pharmacy in the same shopping center. I'm also quite sure they helped keep our family dentist in business as well with access to all that "free" candy. Picture, if you will, Oleson's Mercantile from the hit TV show *Little House on the Prairie*, only most of the time we weren't there buying the right things for the right reasons, and had Nellie been around, she would surely have ended up back at one or many house parties to boot! Hard to believe this was the same Midwest, right?

David and I also shared a mutually strong affection for our dirt bikes, which back in the day were more commonly referred to as "BMX" bikes.

Most people can remember the day they first turned sixteen and couldn't wait to get their driver's license and explore their newfound freedom. For David and me, this day started when we both learned how to kick off the training wheels and explore the world on our bicycles. Nothing screamed "FREEDOM!" to us like the ability to jump on our bikes and go anywhere at any time and for any reason. Bikes also meant that our time at home was largely relegated to sleeping, and only during those nights when we weren't sleeping over at a friend's house instead.

I'm not sure that the current younger generation shares this same feeling, nor do I think most parents today would even allow that level of freedom. Back then, our parents never equipped us with helmets and body pads nor did they give us maps of houses around our neighborhood listing all known sex offenders to avoid on the way to school. I'm pretty sure we thought we could have handled this at the time. Rarely did we ride without strapping a BB gun onto our backs or mounting menacing-looking bottle-rocket launchers from our handlebars, just waiting for our next victim to appear.

David and I spent a lot of time together during the early 1980s after the blend started—much to the chagrin of the local bird, squirrel, and rabbit populations, as well as our neighbors, who would have been wise to invest in house window replacement companies during that time. But nothing taught us how to be bad better than having two older brothers and a sister helping us expand our four-letter-word vocabularies and discovering the magical benefits of beer consumption in front of their highly amused friends. I later heard that one of these friends was so inspired by our childhood antics that, while writing for the hit TV show *Beavis and Butt-Head*, he decided to steal some of our material.

I'm not exactly sure what material, if any, Sam got from us, but I do recall placing fireworks inside the finger holes of bowling balls with David and rolling them down a long hill into heavy traffic . . . long before Beavis and Butt-Head did the same thing. I also remember some pretty nasty BB gun wars, and I'm not talking about the "airsoft" battles you now see kids in with their fully padded-up gear where they can barely feel getting hit. No, these were BB gun wars that would scare the living shit out of parents today . . . including even myself now that I'm a parent.

The first rule in a BB gun war was the "one-pump" rule on our Crosman Pumpmaster 760 BB guns. This rule really only applied to people you were shooting at who were very close friends. Everybody else got more pumps—the more you hated them or wanted to inflict maximum pain, the more pumps they got. At that time, nobody could afford to buy any real body protection, and eye protection was always optional as well. Like I said, this should scare the shit out of any parent reading this.

Now, by this time, David and I had fired so many thousands of rounds through our BB guns that we could have very well qualified for any military sniper school. We were that good! We knew all elevations on our holds out past one hundred yards, how to account for windage, and could reload and rapid-fire better than most kids that day with repeating rifles. This also made us deadly in a BB gun war, and we knew it. For that reason alone, we made sure that we were almost always on the same side of a battle. We were so good at coordinating our attacks that we had defilade and flanking maneuvers down pat before most kids had ever heard of such things in a war movie. But no battle was really complete without the added use of field artillery courtesy of Rock Port, Missouri, fireworks.

Like I mentioned, our older siblings were saints and always looked out for us. This included buying us an infinite supply of illegal fireworks each summer during their road trips from Omaha to Rock Port, Missouri, where class-C fireworks were both legal and always in supply. We would save up all our money and would even borrow some if needed to buy as many gross of bottle rockets, artillery shells, Black Cats, missiles, etc., as we could get our hands on. Half of the loot was used for tormenting the neighborhood throughout the summer while the other half was sold, commonly at double the price, to other kids in the area who either didn't have good connections or didn't have role model older siblings like we did. *Isn't capitalism great?!*

Now, the combination of BB guns and explosives made for a lot of fun, and perhaps the greatest battles of all happened when the city decided to shut down and widen 90th Street in front of our house. We were originally told that the process would take around six months to complete but when it lingered on for over a year, we weren't surprised. For months at a time, the city dug trenches and laid huge pipes and valves throughout the dirt mounts and trenches that had once been our street. It was as if the gods of war descended upon us and said, "Here is the mother of all battlefields and we placed it right in front of your house. Enjoy!" And enjoy we did.

At this point, we were freshly restocked from Rock Port and by now had also learned that flash powder, when carefully removed from hundreds of Black Cat inch-and-a-halfers could be "repurposed" into new devices that I'm quite sure the government would reclassify well above class-C fireworks. We confirmed this fact when testing our new devices on some of the most beautiful and ornate stone mailboxes around the area, resulting in something that would make any supernova jealous. We also found these devices to be useful in prolonging city construction timelines as well.

So now the battlefield was set. We knew the trenches in and out, where to strategically hide artillery and our new "devices," and how to win the battles. All we needed at this point were some French Soldiers to make this look easy, and we found them courtesy of our older siblings' drunken friends. The plan was easy. Get them drunk, hand them a bunch of harmless Roman candles, and then let them think they could win the war by coming after us "little kids." As they would soon find out, no matter how much alcohol you consume, BBs and missiles hurt like hell when they hit you over and over . . . and they continue to hurt the morning after as well. *Ha!*

Now, injuring older drunk teens and delaying city work projects were only a few of our many accomplishments growing up. In the early days, David and I both played on the same soccer team together—David played wing and I played guard. As I continued to play and move on to learn many of the other common seasonal sports in Nebraska, David continued with soccer and was damn good at it. During those first years of the early 1980s, David and I spent a lot of time together. This I would quickly learn would become somewhat unusual for the rest of our family, except for our annual family "vacations" to our family cabin located in Grand Lake, Colorado.

Our week-long trips would always start by loading up our cars, which included an old station wagon that was not far off from the now famous Wagon Queen Family Truckster from the hit movie *National Lampoon's Vacation,* and then waiting what seemed like forever in the driveway for Mom to finally get out to the cars with a coffee cup in hand, necessitating the always avoidable potty stop sixty minutes after departure. One year we decided that our dog Dandy could stay home, so we placed six bowls of dog food and a large barrel of water by the front door and drove away, saying good-bye to our loyal dog. *Why he stuck around is beyond me— he had his chance!*

We then started the journey west across the fruited plains for eleven to twelve hours of driving across a landscape that would make the Flat Earth Society proud. Back then, the government decided to torture us further by limiting the speed limit to 55 miles per hour, which is about as entertaining as watching paint dry. In later years once we were "legal" to drive, we kids decided to set a few land speed records from Omaha to Grand Lake that I'm quite sure were only previously held by aircraft. A few family dinners that followed included pissing contests about who made it there fastest. Eight hours. Even seven hours.

"Impossible . . . no way," responded an uncle who overheard one such conversation about these record driving times. Despite his adamant tone of disbelief, we all just smiled and walked away. I knew the times were true. I was there when we buried the speedometer needle on the car that day and never stopped once for Texas Toast in Julesburg *(Sorry, Joe)* or even to piss—we had plenty of empty beer cans onboard for that.

But early on, before our new speed records, David and I would jump in the rearward-facing seat in the back of the station wagon and away we went, stopping at our usual spots that Clark Griswold must have missed on his way to see the largest ball of twine on the face of the earth. These included traditional stops at such "landmarks" as Buffalo Stuckey's to see their baby rattlers and the Old Jules Café so Joe could get his normal fix of Texas Toast. And nothing was more exciting than, sixty miles into the trip, hearing Joe call out that we were passing the state capitol building in Lincoln, which he affectionately referred to as the "penis of the plains." *Eat your heart out, Clark Griswold.*

Along our journey, David and I decided that any car that came up behind us could see us in the back seat, which we took full advantage of. If they passed us, it was our chance to yell at Joe for driving too slow. If it was a trucker, we always gave the sign to honk their horn. For everybody else, we would show another sign that typically involved one of our five fingers. Care to guess which one?

We were terrible passengers and only made it worse for Joe as he tried to do more than one thing at a time. Joe loved to dictate comments into his portable Dictaphone for his secretary while driving. This was amusing around town for short stretches at a time but was downright torture for passengers stuck in a car listening to it for eleven to twelve hours. So, true to our nature, we decided to make sure Joe was able to get as little work done as possible while with us on these trips. Early on this would result in spankings in the living room, but that didn't last long when David and I would simply laugh at him during the administration process and then tease him after about his weight and lack of stamina in whacking our asses. Did I mention we were also pros at using reverse psychology on people?

Despite these sometimes-tortuous drives to Colorado, we all loved Grand Lake. The place was and still is truly magical and if you have been there, you know what I mean. We stayed at our family cabin, located on the infamous Scout Rock, which sits on fifteen acres and at its peak overlooks Shadow Mountain Lake—the twin lake adjoining Grand Lake. The cabin was built over a hundred years ago, which is probably the last time anybody updated the kitchen in that place. It can sleep up to fourteen people, and when Joe's grandmother Ida purchased it back in 1954 she added two adjoining bathrooms, making the skunk in the outhouse very happy to finally be alone. It was rustic but beautiful. If you could handle the occasional spider bite at night and "Nat the bat" occasionally flying through the living room, the place was about as close to God and nature as one could get while still having running water.

I still cannot spend time at Scout Rock without thinking of David. So many of my childhood memories in Grand Lake involve time spent with David. What made Grand Lake even more magical early on was the fact that many of the kids we knew in the area had just as much of a propensity for getting into trouble as we did—we were right at home! Literally! I mean, the minute we hit the cabin, we unloaded our bikes, loaded our BB guns and we were gone into town to the arcades, into the woods to hike, camp, and fish, and into the property to exterminate the chipmunk population that had survived the previous winter. We had chipmunk hunting down so cold that one year an aunt who visited the cabin after we left made a comment to the family about how strange it was to not see one chipmunk during her trip. And we didn't always need BB guns to make this happen, either. We had plenty of time to think up new ways to hunt, and some of them included cereal.

Chipmunks like to eat—we all do. One year somebody decided to bring up a "regular" box of

Rice Krispies cereal instead of our preferred choice of Frosted Rice Krispies. I mean, come on—why add sugar to a cereal that is already sold pre-sugared? Not to mention that the sugar in the Scout Rock sugar jar was likely as old as the cabinets in the kitchen. So why run the risk? *Sugar expires, right?* So, as always, we kids made the best of a bad situation and decided to feed the unwanted Rice Krispies to the chipmunks . . . over a rat trap, of course.

"Oh my God, did you just see that?!" yelled my brother Doug. "The chipmunk started eating the Rice Krispies at the top of Scout Rock and whoosh, there was a cloud of Rice Krispies everywhere!"

Success! This way of hunting chipmunks was a hell of a lot more effective than using a BB gun! Not to mention the entertainment value alone was worth the effort. But Rice Krispies, BB guns, and bikes were not the only things we brought with us on our trips to Grand Lake. After all, what is summer without fireworks, right? Even up in the high mountains with dry timber and fire bans, what could possibly go wrong? Well, one day we decided to find out with the help of our cousins who decided to stay with us during the trip. And all of this happened on Scout Rock.

As the old stories go, Scout Rock was named for Indian scouts who would sit on the rock overlooking the valley below, which is now flooded to form

Shadow Mountain Lake. One day, a scout fell asleep on the rock, allowing a warring tribe to approach undetected, leading to a slaughter and the eventual launch of the fleeing Indian women and children into canoes across Grand Lake. At that time, a storm struck and sunk the canoes, killing all aboard. So as legend goes, Grand Lake was first named "Spirit Lake" by the Indians, who said the early morning mist over the lake was the spirit of those Indians who died on the lake that day. And all of this apparently started because of a bad decision made on Scout Rock. Well, we kids, along with our cousins, decided to add to the list of dubious achievements on this famous and hallowed land.

It all started with rows and rows of bottle rockets and missiles that were now lined up as far as I could see in a manner that would have made even Napoleon proud. All of the artillery, freshly imported from Rock Port, Missouri, via Omaha was facing in one menacing direction. We had spent an hour or more lining everything up while carefully surveying the flight path of each rocket, which now must have numbered into the many hundreds. *I'm pretty sure I lost count after a while.*

Punks were now lit, with backup punks lit as well. We were ready! And then we heard them, the sound of horseback riders slowly making their way up the road between our property below Scout Rock and Shadow Mountain Lake on the other side. In the military they would refer to this as a perfect "choke point," but the riders would soon call this something else—something I'm pretty sure would involve words not safe for television. Just as the riders reached our ambush point, the fuses were lit and all hell broke loose.

Now, I have heard and seen professional fireworks displays many times, but this was on a whole other level. The peaceful joyride these poor folks paid for turned into something only seen as a bucking bronc riding rodeo. Horses were running everywhere, including into the lake. *Who knew horses didn't like being shot at with fireworks? Hell, we kids were used to it by now.* Our Grand Lake fireworks show was so impressive that I'm surprised they didn't ask us to run the official show over the lake in the years that followed. But they had to catch us first and, once all of the damage was done, we stayed true to the path provided by the Indians before us and got the hell out of there and headed for Grand Lake. *Like I said before, it was amazing we all survived.*

As the years rolled on, we all started to grow our separate ways—even during our trips to Grand Lake. I guess the rentals must have decided that we couldn't do enough damage together as a family so they now decided to let each of us bring along a friend on our trips to Grand Lake. *Brilliant!* We still managed to get into trouble, just not always together. But you could always count on one bond we all shared that continued to bring us back together—beer! Although I could write a whole book on our "doings" in Grand Lake alone, I would be remiss if I didn't at least mention one of my favorite stories . . . which also including fireworks. I know, shocking, right?

Grand Lake was a shared cabin amongst a growing number of family members who all received a week or so to use it during high season in the summer. Because the cabin was never winterized, the high season was often short, leaving only a week or so of really prime time in the mountains before the next family group came along. This system worked out pretty well for quite a while, thanks in large part to the efforts of Uncle Jock, who lived in Denver and was in a perfect place to oversee the cabin throughout the years. Uncle Jock, who we kids affectionately referred to as "Jock strap," was commodore of the Grand Lake Yacht Club and he along with his wife, Nancy, were pretty cool people, I thought. Except for one problem—they didn't seem to like us kids very much. Can you blame them? Hell, if I were them I probably wouldn't like us, either. I'm sure the fact that they didn't have children of their own played into this . . . that, as well as a gross of bottle rockets that went off in the cabin during one of their dinner parties.

"DEDE, this is Betty. You are never going to guess who just called me," she said while laughing over the phone. Betty was Joe's mother and if anybody could appreciate a good practical joke, it was her. I only knew her during the last few years of her life but she was always a sweetheart and I always thought that Joe got many of his best qualities from her. Apparently, my mother must have been in a good mood as well because she couldn't stop laughing herself when she told me the news. And here is what happened.

My friend Colby and I thought it would be funny to stuff a gross of bottle rockets in the flue of the fireplace in the living room of the cabin. For those of you who are unfamiliar with fireworks lingo, a gross is 144 exploding rockets all tightly bound into one package. Because the cabin was not winterized, the fireplace was built to support some monstrous fires when needed and included a large area that a half dozen people could comfortably sit around and even sleep around during those really cold mountain nights. So, we thought by placing these rockets in the flue of the fireplace, they were bound to go off at some point while we were all there. Well, they didn't and we left after a week, forgetting about the gift we unintentionally left for the next family to enjoy. As it turned out, it was Jock; his wife, Nancy; and all of their adult friends who enjoyed a second Fourth of July fireworks display courtesy of us.

Apparently, they were all sitting down for a formal dinner when the entertainment started. Now, 144 exploding rockets can take some time to all go off, so apparently somebody in the entourage had enough time to figure out who must have done this *(Are you surprised?)* and decided to call Grandma Betty to inform them. Betty told Mom that as this person proceeded to yell into the phone at Betty, she could hear the fireworks continuing to go off in the background and had a hard time not laughing during the call. *It must run in the family.*

Eventually all the rockets exploded, the party went on, and our relatives developed a newfound fondness for our side of the family from Omaha. This was a common theme in the extended family that ultimately encouraged the rentals to build a new and modern cabin in Grand Lake some years later, which we now enjoy thoroughly. And yes, our kids have plenty of BB guns to help keep traditions alive, although they don't seem to compare to the new thrill of gaming a whole world-war on their smart phones and then stopping only a few feet away from lunch when it's ready. *At least nobody is shooting their eyes out.* But as much as I continue to remember David on our continued trips to Grand Lake, there was one trip when I was trying my best to forget.

Shortly after David died we all took another family trip to Scout Rock. This was my son Chase's first trip to Grand Lake, but, being so little at the time, he wouldn't remember. My wife did, though, and the sleepless nights with Chase suffering from altitude sickness certainly didn't help her "enjoy" vacation much on that trip. But there was also a somberness on this trip because a member of our family was now gone. We all took a family picture on Scout Rock and you can still tell by looking at our faces that something was missing. My sister, Amy, made this painfully clear to me one morning during that same trip.

"Hey, Dust, do you want to join me in scattering some of David's ashes near Adams Falls this afternoon?" *Holy shit! Amy still had some of David's ashes with her?* I was so caught off guard by her request that I initially didn't know how to react. *What happened to finding closure and moving on? Do I really want to relive David's burial all over again?* So, I responded in the only way I knew how at the time.

"I'm sorry, Amy, but I cannot go through burying David all over again. I hope you understand that I need closure with his loss," I said to my sister. She seemed a little stunned by my response. Much like my own reaction to her request, she didn't seem to know how to initially respond back to me. *Now this is really awkward.* After a brief pause, she responded as respectfully as possible.

"I understand and certainly didn't want you to feel uncomfortable," she said. "I just know how much you and David loved Grand Lake, so I thought we could leave some of his ashes here."

Amy was right; I should have gone with her. But after losing my father at a young age, I had learned to convince myself to harden up when it came to death and that there was a time to mourn and after that, you needed to move on. In my mind, this was called closure and with it came a recalcitrant desire to move forward and not dwell on past losses, especially when it came to losing family members. But as I would learn in the years to follow, closure with David would not come at the burying of his ashes. As much as I regret not going with my sister that day, my time and closure with David was far from over, and no hardening of my mind could change that.

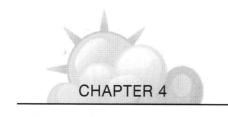

CHAPTER 4

KINDRED SPIRITS

"Dusty, did you see this coming? You and David were so close," my sister, Amy, asked.

I looked back at Amy with a curious stare. *Who, me?* I thought to myself. *I was David's stepbrother. Surely Amy had a better read on him then I did, right?* Or so I thought.

"No, I had no idea there was even a problem," I responded to Amy. "I don't remember David even mentioning a problem or suicide." In hindsight, that was only partially true. I do remember a much younger David in his early teens who did mention suicide, but that was many years ago now and surely we had outgrown those kinds of thoughts, I had quietly thought to myself. Clearly, I was wrong. There was obviously something there that never quite went away. But why now and not then? What finally triggered David to actually do what I always discounted as a crude and veiled threat in our youth to get more attention? *What did I miss? Hindsight is 20/20.*

As the years progressed growing up together, David and I started coming into our own and separate lives. David become an artist and also enjoyed "things" beyond just alcohol. I followed my inner cowboy and decided to build and race NASCAR at the unusually young age of fifteen. Now, smoking pot and stock car racing go together like oil and water, so even though we would occasionally cross paths at local parties, life marched on and it seemed like our lives were forever growing our own ways except for the one thing we both always mutually loved that helped bring us back together.

David went away to college at Northern Arizona University (NAU) to pursue a degree in art a year before I graduated from high school. NAU is located in the northern Arizona mountain town of Flagstaff, and if you like outdoor mountain life without always freezing your ass off, then Flagstaff could very well be the heaven that still eludes you. But I, like most people at the time, didn't know much of anything about Flagstaff. *It's in Arizona, right? What part of the desert is it in?*

Flagstaff was the last college I looked at and ironically it happened after I had already initially registered as a freshman at Colorado State University. It was a last-minute trip to Flagstaff and after that I was hooked. Two hours to the south I could live my early childhood dream of being a cowboy and, up north, I could ski in the winter and live in a mountain region that in many ways resembled the Colorado mountains I grew up around. What more could I want? My fears of possibly becoming homesick were also eased knowing that David would be in the same town with me for at least three of the next few years. *Back together again.*

As it turned out, I wasn't ready for college then and a full year in Flagstaff proved this point. While most kids were going to classes, I decided to major in my fraternity and minor in outdoor adventures and partying. *Nine months of college down the drain!* During this time of eternal bliss and a scholastic record that would make Bluto from *Animal House* proud, I did have something that I did responsibly on a weekly basis, and it involved David.

Every Sunday David and I would meet for breakfast at a local greasy spoon called Choi's, which was famous for their $2.99 steak and eggs breakfast. Even though three bucks was manageable for poor college folks like us, we would have paid more for the time spent together. *It was worth it!* I would share stories with David about how my fraternity seemed to be writing the book on how hazing could get you well past double-secret probation and David would tell me about his hippie friends and the alternative art world. We also talked about our family and laughed at all the crazy stories of growing up together. These breakfast meetings meant more to me than David probably ever knew and ultimately led to even more priceless moments together.

One of these happened when David invited me over to his apartment near NAU to hang out with him and his hippie friends. I'm always up for some good reverse psychology humor so I decided to dress up and wear shoes for the occasion, which removed any potential doubt as to who was the white elephant in the room that day. Now, I'm not quite sure how I managed to get a reprieve that night from my usual fraternal hazing but I'd certainly had enough Sunday night lineups and nude runs through sorority houses at that point to earn a night off. I later learned that my fraternity was eventually kicked off campus for hazing. My only response when I heard the news was, "What took them so long?"

The party turned out to be everything I thought it would be. I felt like one of those people at the end of *Close Encounters of the Third Kind* who were surrounded by the aliens that were curiously touching a human for the first time. Only in this case, I was the foreign creature and had clearly landed smack dab in the middle of modern-day Woodstock. I'm not sure many of these people had ever really sat down and talked to a diehard capitalist pig before, so I decided to have a little fun with this one. By the end of the night, I was the only person not high as a kite, which allowed me to creatively freak out some of these people with tales of hazing and capitalism that included just a hint of embellishment for fun. *Too bad I didn't record this.* Shortly after the "party," family called.

Our sister, Amy, decided she was going to get married in Omaha, which led to our next adventure together. We both jumped into my truck and drove down to Phoenix to catch a flight back to Omaha for the festivities and the debauchery—which we decided to get an early start on. I mean, why wait for the fun to start when we already had a plane stocked full of booze to keep us busy at thirty thousand feet, right? So, we managed to bribe the flight attendant to serve us an unlimited number of drinks on the plane ride home, which was impressive for two kids who weren't even of legal age to drink at all—let alone on a commercial flight. By the time we got off the plane, well, Amy later told us that we did a great job of barely stumbling off the jetway after we landed. The party proceeded as planned and the night ended with a full round of mailbox baseball with my buddies who never left home. *Just like old times!*

Now, I had a few friends in Omaha who liked to let bad habits die hard and I certainly wasn't going to disappoint them during my sister's wedding weekend back home. So, after a sobering flight and the parties that followed at the downtown bars, we decided that all those beautiful, ornate mailboxes around our old neighborhood that were somehow spared during our "explosive" youth needed a little work. Making matters worse was that this night of all nights was "trash night" in Omaha, when people would bring out their cans to the street in front of their houses for pickup the next morning. We decided to help them get started early with this.

So, we jumped into Kyle's car, which, like all of Kyle's old cars, would never pass a modern-day inspection test to be deemed even remotely street-legal. Now, just prior to our departure, my friends who were already inebriated told our father, Joe, that they would be there first thing tomorrow morning to help drive people to the wedding services. *Joe should have known better than to even ask.* So off we went on a night's outing that led me to seriously question whether or not I could actually die from laughing too hard. *It's a good thing I went away to get a higher education.*

The next morning started with a good tongue lashing from Joe.

"Where the hell are your friends?! They told me they would be here to help drive people to the wedding!" Joe yelled in utter disbelief. Now, I'm not sure exactly when Joe thought that my old friends would become responsible people, but he was the only person surprised that morning.

"Joe, maintain an even strain," I replied while making a few phone calls that I knew would go unanswered. In the end, we all managed to get to the wedding on time and when I later asked Kyle what happened, he told me that after dropping me off that night, the police managed to track down his car and made him and the others go back and fix all the damage they caused that night. Kyle told me that they knew I had the wedding in the morning so they didn't want to make me join them. *Thanks, Kyle—I still owe you one!* Once again, we all managed to survive, and then David and I headed back to Flagstaff together.

But one of our final and perhaps most important times together in Arizona happened one weekend in Flagstaff when I received a totally unexpected call from David.

"OK, Roo, come on over and pick me up. I am taking you up on your offer." One of my nicknames was "Roo," which David used often. We had many nicknames growing up, some of which are not safe to print, but Roo was mine and seemed to stick with David. It all started when we first blended as a family and David and I decided that we both loved the Winnie-the-Pooh characters Tigger and Roo. As usual, I was the youngest member of the clan, so naturally the youngest character fit me well. But despite the name, this call was totally out of left field and was one I never thought I would receive. And it all had to do with his hair.

David grew out his hair years ago for a musical he'd starred in called—what else?—*Hair*. Since that time, he seemed to take his role literally and, along with the hippie counterculture of the day, it seemed to stick. Not only that; it grew out in epic proportions, always giving me good ammo on David every time I saw him, which eventually led to a promise I never thought he would eventually take me up on.

At the time of the call I still couldn't believe it! Over the years, David had grown out this long and mangy mop of hair that could have hidden any bird's nest from plain sight. I guess it was part of the hippie culture and David took a lot of pride in it—without much maintenance and cleaning, to boot. I had always joked with David that any time he wanted to cut his hair, I would pay for it. And what do you know, today was the day. I honestly had never thought this day would come, so I was still in disbelief.

So, we drove over to Supercuts, which was probably the only place that would have considered this cut, and when David sat down in the chair, the barber didn't even know where to start. Neither did I, but I promised him a well-earned tip once he was done.

"Just cut it all off and cut it short," David said. *Holy cow, what will his Woodstock friends think when they see this?* Would they blame his fascist capitalist brother for corrupting him? I started to have serious reservations about this, but David had made up his mind and I wasn't about to renege on my offer. By the time the barber was done, the floor looked like a fire hazard and I still expected a bird or two to fly out from it. The hair was gone and my brother David started to look like the kid I grew up with back in Omaha again. So, we decided to celebrate.

After leaving the barber shop, we picked up a case of beer and drove down to the Verde River, where under a beautiful sky we proceeded to drink and wade through the river for hours on end, telling funny stories and talking about our crazy family back home. It was such a great day and hard to really describe—*you almost had to be there to really understand it.* The abruptness of David's call. The suddenness of him wanting to cut off his long hair. The trip down to the Verde River to drink and reflect together. It was at this time that I finally came to the realization that David was more than just my stepbrother. He was a kindred spirit.

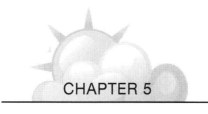

CHAPTER 5

THE CALLING

"Oh my God, I can't move my body," I said, lying catatonic in my bed next to my wife. I have always heard stories of people getting "their calling" or "their awakening" in life and I thought I had just received mine . . . even though it came wrapped in a riddle.

"What's wrong?" my wife Joanie asked as I suddenly woke her up from her sleep.

"I can't believe what just happened to me," I said, still lying motionless in our bed. "I still can't move my body. You are never going to believe what just happened to me," I said, still in shock and disbelief after the minute or two that would end up changing my life forever.

At that time Joanie and I were living in a two-bedroom, two-bath apartment in Dunwoody, Georgia, a close-in suburb of Atlanta, where we both worked. The apartment was designed with a kitchen and living room running through the middle of the apartment, leaving a bedroom and bath on either side. We were young, in our mid-twenties and just starting out our lives together. I had first met Joanie when we were fixed up by my sister and brother-in-law, Cliff, during a fun weekend getaway to their former home in Novi, Michigan, a suburb of Detroit.

My trips to hang out and party with Amy and Cliff first started after my graduation from college. Prior to that our interactions were largely limited to "nights out" in Omaha and Lincoln, where Cliff and I would always manage to shock and offend everyone around us with our constant but friendly physical abuse of each other in public. It was a rare night out with Cliff when the pain of a hangover the day after could compete with a good kidney punch or head-butt the night before. One of my favorite moments like this happened during a night out together in Omaha when we all decided to have dinner at a formal restaurant in the Flatiron Hotel. Being the true boneheads that we were together, we decided to make a grand entrance that night.

Cliff was the first one through the door, which happened to be in full view of most of the patrons there that evening for what they surely thought was going to be a nice and quiet night out. Once through the door, I gave Cliff a kidney shot that even Mike Tyson would have been proud of. Cliff yelled and dropped to his knees while managing to get off a quick kick backward that perfectly nailed me in the family jewels. We both dropped to the floor in agony while everybody in the restaurant stopped eating and looked our way in total disbelief. Now, I had seen my sister, Amy, mad before, but this was a new level of anger and disgust and a shade of red I had never seen on her face. We were out of there so fast that I'm quite sure they were happy to cancel our reservation. But the fun continued after college as well.

The summer after my college graduation involved a trip to see Cliff and Amy at their home at the time in Cincinnati. Both of them were working during the days so we partied at night, which included watching Cliff eat enough ghost chilies, causing the chefs at certain restaurants to actually come out to see if he was still alive. And during the days, well, I hit the pool and watched enough reruns of *Dumb and Dumber* to memorize every line. We always had a great time on these trips, so Amy and Cliff thought they would "surprise" me during another trip to see them in Michigan by setting me up with one of their friends and coworkers, Joanie, who was now living in Atlanta. We hit it off that weekend and shortly after I returned home to Omaha, I decided to quit my job and move to Atlanta to join her. She thought I was nuts for making such an impetuous decision, but I knew what I wanted and, since football season was over in Nebraska, it was time to make my move.

We first moved to an area called Buckhead, which at the time was the party capital of Atlanta—and the whole south, for that matter. Atlanta was a great city to start out in. It was affordable, the weather was good, the people were friendly, and they were rabid college football fans, so I fit right in. After a short time in Buckhead, we moved to the next area over, called Dunwoody, where we rented a larger apartment closer to work. If you've ever driven in Atlanta traffic, you know how important this is. Everything seemed to be "normal" until that night happened and changed everything.

Now, I've heard people talk about "out of body" experiences before, but never really paid any attention to it. In my mind, things such as this were interesting but always received with a high level of skepticism. Remember—I was a capitalist pig in the eyes of David's friends, so what did I know? But what I experienced that night changed my views on many things in my life. And it all started with an unexpected journey to our spare bathroom.

It was the middle of the night and out of the blue I found myself moving from my bedroom, through the living room, and through the door to our spare bathroom. Now, normally if I had to get up in the middle of the night—which sadly now happens more often with age—I am half-awake and trying to remember not to miss when I reach the toilet. But this trip was different. I was 100 percent conscious and instead of "finding my way" in the dark I was being pulled through the doorway of our spare bathroom.

Apparently, whoever thought of this journey did one hell of the temporary remodeling job to our spare bathroom, which I was soon to discover. *Who says God doesn't have a sense of humor?* As the door to the bathroom opened I found myself in a large room with a very bright light ahead of me that would have been blinding to the naked eye in the conventional sense but instead was calming and easy to look at. In front of me was a line of pews one would normally see in a church, all facing toward the light, and one lone man sitting in the front pew. I couldn't see his face as he was facing forward with his head slightly down, but from the backside he looked a lot like somebody I used to know. *Was this my father, who I lost when I was six years old?*

As I stood in the back of the room, I heard a voice speak out from what seemed like beyond the light in a deep and authoritative voice. "Stop wasting your talents," the voice said. And that was it. At that point, I was pulled backward from the room, through the living room, and back into the bedroom, where my body remained on the bed where I last left it. As I settled back into my body, I suddenly awoke feeling a sensation all over that I had never felt before. It's still hard to describe this feeling even today other than to say that my body tingled all over and I simply could not move—nor did I want to. My body felt so strange and amazing for the minutes that followed that I began to wonder if this was the "high" David's hippie friends use to tell me I was missing when I decided to "stick with my beer."

As you can imagine, I have struggled with and reflected on this moment in time since that day and continue to question myself as a result: What are the talents that he spoke of that I was apparently wasting, and what is my purpose in life? What I have never questioned, however, was what happened that night and what it meant to me. I know what a dream is and this was not like any dream I have ever experienced. Not even close. What further confirmed this for me was the continued "experiences" I would have that would one day include David—years after this event first took place.

Being the natural skeptic that I am of all things "unnatural," I was hoping that perhaps this was in fact a crazy aberration in my life and would eventually go away. But it didn't, as my wife Joanie and I discovered a short time later during a trip to Detroit to visit Amy and Cliff. We were sleeping in a hotel room when I suddenly woke up and looked over at the chair across the room from the bed. For a brief moment, I saw an older woman sitting there looking at us with an almost emotionless expression on her face. Then I heard her say, "Take care of my little girl."

Now, many people of my generation had their parents read them books before they went to sleep. One of the books that was read to me as a child, oddly enough, was entitled *There's a Nightmare in My Closet*. For those millennials and younger reading this, yes, our parents were skilled at scaring the crap out of us at all the wrong times. Now, I grew up like most people, thinking that if I ever saw something "ghostly" at night in my bedroom, I would dive under the covers and scare myself to sleep. Most people are still this way at any age, if they're being honest that is. That is our natural "emotional" response to the unknown that may scare us. But my emotional reaction to what I witnessed that night was far different then even I would have expected from myself.

"Joanie, what did your favorite grandmother look like?" I asked. "You know, the one you used to talk about with your mother." With this question, I once again woke my wife up from her sleep. *By now she must think I am crazy or something.*

"Why, what happened?" she replied.

At that point I had to try to explain, again, what had just happened to me, only this time I brought someone else very close to my wife into the conversation. After telling her what happened she started asking me questions about what she looked like and what she said. I described her in as much detail as possible. As for what she said to me, well, nobody seems to want to have lengthy conversations with me during these events, so there was not much more to add here. Except for one detail—how the experience "felt" when it happened.

At no time from when the event began did I ever feel the least bit scared. In fact, I felt quite the opposite and certainly not how I would have naturally felt in any other setting. As odd as this may sound, it was almost a pleasant and peaceful experience that left me feeling good as a result. My wife, on the other hand, did not share the same sentiments and wanted to know more. Months later, on one of our many trips back to New York to see her family, she showed me a picture of her grandmother. *Clearly, she didn't want to let this go.*

"Yup, that's her," I said, quickly acknowledging the picture of the same unsmiling woman from that night in the hotel room. The look on Joanie's face told me that it might have been better if I had just kept my mouth shut about the whole event. Sadly, this would be the same problem I would struggle with for years to come after David's death, when other strange things started to happen.

"Do you think it was just a coincidence and she looked like somebody else?" I asked my wife, trying to downplay the whole event in her mind.

"I don't think so," she replied. "She used to refer to me as *her little girl* and almost never had a smile on her face—just like you described."

As the years passed, so, too, did our marriage. After producing two beautiful children together, seven years was apparently all we could make work together, leading to a new chapter in my life. *Yes, I have heard of the seven-year itch. Apparently, it is alive and well in my world.* It took me years to mentally recover from my divorce. Coming to the realization that I would not be able to live with and raise my kids under the same roof every day literally made me ill and took a lot to come to grips with. Growing up, I had heard that my father was "super dad," and that was always my goal—I wanted to be "super dad" for my children, and now that that dream had come crashing down. *What would my dad have thought of me now?* It was one of the lowest points of my life and took years to recover from.

But prior to our separation and inevitable divorce, my "experiences" expanded beyond both my wife's grandmother and my formerly remodeled spare bathroom in Dunwoody to include somebody much closer to me, somebody I thought I had reached closure with on August 25, 2002, when I did what I always tried to do: cry, mourn, see them put to rest, and then attempt to move on with life. As I would soon learn, life is not that simple and the lessons I should have learned during my moment in the spare bathroom years prior were coming back to me full force. It also became painfully apparent to me that I was not seeking these things out—they were finding me. *But why? I am the last person to want to believe any of this was real.*

Now, before I begin telling about my experiences with David, I want to start with a clear disclaimer here. There are many different teachings about and interpretations of what happens to people when they die. Many people believe that you ascend to a heaven while others believe that your greatest contributions from that point on come from pushing up daisies. There are further and more foggy teachings and beliefs amongst the "heaven can wait crowd" about what happens when you end your life by suicide. Do you go straight to heaven? Do you go to hell? Or do you go somewhere in between? I am not going to attempt to answer any of these questions based on what I believe or want to believe. Yes, I do have my own personal beliefs and I have always considered myself to be a spiritual person with less allegiance to formalized religion. But in a world filled with 7.5 billion people practicing thousands of different religions, I would prefer to stick with what I have experienced and let the theologians of the world preach and pontificate their own religious meaning of it. At the end of this story I will share my own meaning to all of this but, again, that part is based on what I believe. Now to what I experienced . . . .

Growing up can be a challenging and confusing process—especially when your dreams while sleeping mess with the reality you are trying to learn from when awake. As we grow older, we seem to be better able to distinguish between the two. Yet we still seem to "lose control" of our actions, outcomes, and decisions we make when we dream. Only when we wake afterward do we say to ourselves, "What the hell was I thinking when I did that?" or, if it was a bad dream, "Thank God that ended!" Any of this sound familiar? To me, a dream is now easy to distinguish from anything else because I cannot control my situation, my actions, and my conscious reactions to them while dreaming. I came to this conclusion when I started experiencing something else.

My first experiences with David started in my sleep when I thought I was just having terrible nightmares about the haunting death of my brother. Because of this, I initially spared my wife the further nightly wake-up calls. *Why make our divorce happen any quicker, right?* But they seemed to continue and in very odd ways. Instead of losing control in a dream, I was able to consciously think through these interactions to the point where I could stop and ask questions in a way I could only do when I was awake. So, they continued until one night when I had to say something to Joanie.

"David doesn't know that he is dead," I told her, knowing that I was once again clearly walking out of our comfort zone.

"What do you mean?" she replied. That's when I spilled the beans about the haunting nights I'd had with David up to that point. Many of these encounters involved places I was familiar with while others involved places I would soon become acquainted with after the fact. One of these new places of note was David's old house in La Pine, Oregon, which he lived in with some of his friends for a few years after college. I had never visited or seen pictures of this place prior to these experiences, but there I was, running through the pine trees and streams with David, just like old times. But it was not like old times in La Pine, and only when I was finally able to find an old picture of the house a year or so later did I clearly see in print exactly what I had seen in my own "experiences"—down to the detail. *OK—now this is definitely not a dream!*

In all of my time spent with David, we seemed to be doing all the outdoor things that we loved to do together, but he never once seemed to show any emotion while doing them. It was almost as if he was simply "going through the motions" with me. *This was really odd!* Why was I able to enjoy my time with David again and even express my joy with him while he couldn't even respond with a simple smile or a simple sign of the joy I used to see on his face throughout our childhood while doing the same things? That is when I knew something was really off, and the fact that I was conscious of this problem during these experiences made it even more painful. And that is when I decided to consciously do something to try to help.

During one of our many runs together in the woods, I decided to stop David and sit him down. His face and his reactions were as they always were now—confused and emotionless. His face was like our surroundings—beautiful but always grey and gloomy. It was as if we both became color blind together in a place devoid of sunlight. Now, I had heard jokes about the lack of sunlight in the Pacific Northwest, but this was way beyond that. I'd experienced enough shitty rainy days in New York City alone to know the difference.

"David, do you know that you are dead?" I asked, while looking him straight in the face. Once again, no emotion was given, just a look of confusion. "Why are you running around here like you aren't?" I asked him. Again, more confusion, as if he had no idea what I was even telling him. I might as well have been speaking Chinese to him—it simply didn't compute for David. It was clear to me at that point that he was lost and needed help. *Now what the hell do I do? Does anybody have the phone number for the Ghostbusters?* Seriously, though—who the hell do I call now to figure this all out? What was I supposed to do? And why did he keep coming back to me instead of haunting somebody else?

This was all going on at a time when things were really getting difficult for me. I had just separated from my wife, going through the hell that was my other reality of now living without my children full time. I had moved into a small rental house located near my kids and my ex-wife and had just started a new job. I was also single for the first time in nearly a decade and clearly had no game—nor was I emotionally ready for a serious relationship at that point, so it was probably just as well. *You mean you can now find women online? Who knew?* But things were about to get worse.

By now I had many months of "experiences" with David and it was only recently that I started having my "Come to Jesus" conversations with him when we were together. I could tell he was starting to get even more confused the more I brought this up, but I had to do something. Now, at this point, I didn't know who to call and I certainly wasn't about to tell my friends and family about this. First off, nobody wants to tell their parents and siblings that their son and brother they lost years ago to a tragic suicide may now be living a tragic existence below the pearly gates above. I had seen my stepfather, Joe, tortured enough since David's death and could never spring this on him. The poor guy was just starting to recover and I loved him too much to ever see him lapse back into this world of "what ifs" again.

Secondly, I didn't want people to think I had somehow lost my marbles and needed to be locked up in the looney bin. Remember, I was a capitalist pig who wanted to live a more conventional life free of drugs and problems. I was a businessman at heart, which is something I discovered after nearly flunking out of college my first year as a poli-sci major and then being scholastically reborn into the world of my business college at the University of Nebraska— Lincoln. All it took was taking a class called Personal Finance 201 and I was hooked. Moreover, in college I learned nothing about spiritual encounters while learning the models of the time value of money.

Finally, I simply didn't know anything about why these experiences were happening to me or who could best answer this question. I once asked my ex-wife, but she couldn't help, either. She was born and raised in an Irish-Catholic family, so most of her suggestions began and ended with, "Have you tried calling the Catholic Church?" *Now, why would I do that?* I wasn't a Catholic and two events in particular helped to solidify that her former desire to convert me would never be fulfilled. The first experience happened while attending our first Catholic Church service with her family in New York. Joanie's mother was a devoted Catholic and therefore followed the rules. One of these rules, as I was quick to discover that day, was that non-Catholics were not allowed to take communion in the Catholic Church.

So, as the pews started to empty from front to back to take communion, Joanie's mother said something to her that she passed along to me.

"What are you doing?" she asked, while looking at me inquisitively.

"Well, I'm going to take communion," I responded.

"You're not allowed to take communion in the Catholic Church. Why don't you stay here until we return?" she told me, while I could see her mother listening along agreeingly from her other side.

Now, I have never liked to be told what to do, especially when it made little sense to me why. After all, I was confirmed in the Church of Christ as a child, where I took communion and later did the same at the Barker family's Episcopal church in Omaha. *What the hell?! Why was I the bad guy here?* So, I kept quiet and when the pew before us spilled out and everybody in our pew stood up, I did the only thing I thought was right. I stood up and followed the family up front to take communion. I could tell by the looks from my wife and her mother-in-law along the way that I was in trouble. So, we did our thing and returned to our seats, and that is when she confronted me.

"Why did you take communion? I told you that you were not allowed to in the Catholic Church," she said while I could see her mother listening in from the other side. That was when I decided to explain myself in the only way I knew how and just loudly enough for both my wife and her mother to hear.

"Well, I thought about what you said and here is how I see it. If Jesus Christ were sitting up in the front of the church and saw me walking toward communion, do you think he would have looked at me and said, 'Dustin, sit down. You're not Catholic and cannot take communion before me'?" At that point, well, I had made my point. My wife and her mother, although frustrated, where not prepared to give an answer to my question, so silence was the answer. On a lighter note, my father-in-law, Charlie, apparently overheard this conversation as well and simply looked over and cracked a smile at me.

Now, in all fairness to my wife and her family, they are wonderful people and I knew they were just doing what they were taught by the Church. As best as I could tell, there were no lingering hard feelings about that event, but they clearly understood by my actions and words that I have a slightly different interpretation of religion then they do. And as you will see, this was not the last time I would question some aspects of the Catholic Church.

The second experience happened when the local Catholic Diocese, which included our church, was rocked by the national news of child sexual abuse. During these periods of reported abuse, our two young children were attending the Catholic school affiliated with our church, and when our parish priest decided to go AWOL for services immediately following the breaking news, I was not a happy camper. Now, I hope that nothing bad happened in our church and to the children in the school, but I simply don't know—there was nothing reported that I was aware of. That being said, over the years I have worked closely with attorneys who have handled litigation around these cases and, based on what they told me, many of these abuses and settlements are handled quietly, so we may never really know. However, what I did know after these events was that any remaining chance of me ever joining the Catholic Church was now gone, and since our marriage would not last much longer after that time, it had become a moot point.

Now that my wife and I were apart, nobody else knew about my "experiences." And I had nobody else to confide in except, of course, David. That is until one night at home when everything changed for the worse. I was lying alone in bed when I awoke and heard a voice say to me, "Somebody wants to see you" in a voice as clear and calm as the one I'd heard from my wife's grandmother years before in our Detroit hotel room. At this point I was wide-awake and my life seemed to be in pieces anyways, so I thought, "What the hell; what could possibly happen now?" That was when I discovered what could really go wrong.

Just as I responded "Okay" a huge pulse of energy seemed to slam into my gut, literally knocking me flat on my bed. I literally couldn't move. The energy then spread throughout my body from the tips of my toes to the top of my head. And then came the worst part . . . the feeling of misery and despair like I had never felt before. Now, I had experienced some pretty horrible feelings in my life, but this was on a whole other level. I was crying and screaming and literally felt like I was going to die. Only I quickly realized that these were not my feelings, but rather the feelings of somebody else. *Holy shit—is somebody inside me!?*

After only a minute of this, which felt like an eternity, I couldn't take it anymore. I seriously felt like I was going to die right then and there of sheer despair, so I yelled, "Enough—get out now!" and then the energy once again seemed to condense back into my gut and then pulled away as quickly as it arrived. *Oh my God, what the hell just happened to me?!* Now I was getting scared as I slowly recovered in my bed from what would have made *The Texas Chain Saw Massacre* feel like child's play. This was no longer just a problem, and as I would continue to learn, I couldn't handle this again.

More nights passed and the voice once again woke me up saying, "Somebody wants to see you."

At this point my answer was firmly "NO!" and it continued to obey. During one of the nights that followed I stupidly relented, thinking this must be all my imagination. "Okay," I answered, and once again I felt the pulse of energy hit my gut. "No—get out now!" I quickly yelled before it could get any worse. And that is when I discovered that not only was this not a one-time aberration but that I was somehow able to make it go away as well.

Whatever was creating this energy blast could clearly understand demands, and that is when I learned how to control this and ultimately start shutting it out of my life all together. *Who could be so hopelessly miserable yet also so obediently polite? And was this the same entity politely asking and responding to me or was this something else?* Strange—I could never quite figure this out. But what was much less of a mystery to me was who wanted to visit me, for the timing seemed like no coincidence at all.

Now that I seemed to have these unwanted misery shots in the gut under control, it was time to do what I could during my other nightly experiences. And if my suspicion was correct, both problems could be remedied at the same time. I also added a heavy dose of daily prayers by asking for the same thing that I now forcefully demanded of David in the nights to come.

"David, you are dead and need to go to the heaven," I said over and over again while staring him straight in his face. *No more Mr. Nice Guy. This was starting to get really serious now.* In response, he continued to give me a confused and blank stare. *More Mandarin Chinese, I guess. Maybe I am doing this all wrong. After all, I'm not sure he ever believed in God and heaven to begin with. Time to try something he may better understand and believe in instead.*

"David, you need to find the light and go to it." *Surely, he knew what light was. It would have been damn hard to miss it in the world of grey he kept pulling me into.* I continued with these directions and never gave up. *Between the prayers and the demands somebody had to be listening, right?* It was all I could do. And for some reason he seemed to finally be listening. *But could he understand? Is this why he came to me to begin with? Or did somebody else send him to me instead?* He couldn't seem to talk back, so all I had to go off of was his body language and actions, and something seemed to be telling me that it might be working. *Progress—finally!* But there was only one way I could truly know and that would be if all of this would finally stop.

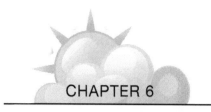

WHY ARE WE HERE?

"Don't give up the fight to stay
alive and even if you have to

Find the reason of another's
pain if they lose you

If not for yourself then
those around who care like I do

One day you'll see the clear blue"

—311, "Beyond the Gray Sky"

"Why am I here?" seems to be the million-dollar
question people have been asking themselves since
the beginning of time. It seems like a logical question
to me. Throughout history the origins and/or
evolution of man has been a hotly debated topic. In
my own world, some argue that man evolved from
apes while others blame Adam and Eve for eating
bad fruit. But what has always amazed me in all this

debate is NOT how we got here, but rather why we are here at all?

I've always loved history and still read a steady flow of history books to keep trying to answer the questions in my own mind about why we are here. If humans are truly doomed to repeat history as so many claim, then certainly there must be a pattern in our madness that we have seen before. In truth, we humans seem to be an enigma by our very nature, and if God truly created us in his own image as many believe, then I always wondered if he had one hell of a sense of humor watching us below for so long. I mean, who needs reality TV when you have 7.5 billion characters all acting below for you?

In my forty-eight years now living on this earth, life to me is full of an endless number of questions and very few profound answers. The night that I was pulled into the ultimate riddle of my life and told to "stop wasting your talents" seems like a microcosm of my life in general. *Now go down there for seventy years and report back on what you learned while I am watching everything you do. And oh, by the way, here are your instructions . . . in four words.* Like I said, God must have one hell of a sense of humor.

In my time here I have also learned a lot about human nature and how we never seem to overcome our own shortcomings. For example, why do we habitually seem to crave what we don't have? Why do we take for granted what we do have? And why don't we always make the right choices when we know what we may do instead is wrong? In my previous books, I have written at length about the effects of "The Contrast Principle" as it pertains to people's behaviors within the business world, but I believe it equally applies to how we live and view our lives as well.

The whole principle is rather simple and is based on the idea that the decisions we make in and about our lives are based on our experiences we can contrast them with. This means that our perceptions of things involving cost, size, worth, value, appearance, and even life are related to and affected by the exposure and stimulus received from comparable others we experience both before and after. And it is these comparable others that ultimately allow us to "know" if what we are buying, doing, evaluating, seeing, experiencing, and even loving is relatively good or not. So being a capitalist businessman, I always prefer to start with the simple numbers.

When it comes to really "appreciating what you have," sometimes the numbers alone can be convincing. Consider this: Of the approximately 7.5 billion people in the world today, 326 million are fortunate enough to be living in the United States (a 1 in 23 chance). Of those living in the US, nearly one-third, or 100 million US citizens, are living at or near the poverty line. This means that there is only a 1 in 33 chance of ever living in the US above the poverty line. Is that you? Now, if you believe in reincarnation as many people do and you live above the poverty line in the US, then your odds of returning to a similar or better situation after you die is only 1 in 33. And if you don't believe in reincarnation, well, what if you're wrong? What are the odds of that? Certainly a lot better than landing on your feet again in the good old US of A. But the numbers alone can't tell the whole story.

I have always believed that by nature we don't know and truly don't appreciate what we want until we know what we don't. These lessons really started for me in my early teens, when I discovered what it was like to do shit work and get paid minimum wage for doing it. This seems to be an experience an increasing number of youth today do not share with the previous generations, so it is worth pointing out here in my own life experiences.

One of these first experiences was working as a busboy at a local fried chicken joint in Omaha. Ironically, my family had eaten there a time or two prior to my taking the job, but once I saw what I saw working there, well, that was the last time I ever ate there. As busboys, we spent nearly all of our time doing the work that nearly everybody else didn't want to do. This primarily included cleaning off tables and dirty dishes and then resetting the tables for the next guests.

Now, even childhood logic told me that when somebody is done with their plate in a restaurant, the remaining food goes into the trash. But I had a classy manager who tried to teach me otherwise. In this case, we were instructed that any uneaten roll or biscuit was to be "returned" to the bin for further serving. Now, I know what you're probably thinking right now but, like I said, I never ate there again and fortunately this restaurant closed a long time ago. But the only person who I felt had it worse than us was the poor guy washing the dishes, who took the bus from downtown Omaha to work every day. He was twice my age and I will never forget watching him run a small bead of water across the top of his cigarettes to make them burn longer. He once told me he did this because he couldn't afford to smoke any other way. This was something I never saw my friends do, for they never needed to—most of them had an allowance that paid for these death sticks.

My second shit job for minimum wage came when I worked on the grounds crew at a large sports and entertainment complex in Omaha call AKSARBEN (that's Nebraska spelled backward . . . catchy, isn't it?). Anyway, on my first day on the job I was handed a Weedwacker, a can of gas, and a jug of water and then dropped off for the rest of the day in a desolate field full of knee-high grass and weeds. And there I stayed, cutting weeds and grass for eight hours with bloodier shins than I ever saw playing guard in a soccer game. *I swear I can still hear that damn Weedwacker buzzing in my ear now.*

The grounds manager who hired me for this job later told me that this was his way of determining if a new hire was tough enough to work there. Apparently, this was an effective process for weeding out new workers (no pun intended), as witnessed by the surprised looks on their faces when I unexpectedly returned for work the next day. Clearly, he had no idea what I had seen prior to this job and I am quite certain I highly recommended a certain fried chicken joint for him to visit after the fact, just to thank him for his hospitality. These were some of the foundational moments when I learned what I didn't want in my work life.

But some of my greatest life lessons about the value of the Contrast Principle also came from people who had seen and experienced a much different and much less fortunate life than I have or would ever experience at minimum wage. The first of these came from my grandfather George, who in many respects was like a second father to me both before and after the death of my own father. I spent a lot of quality time with George growing up, and we had a lot in common. We both liked to hunt together, build things, travel, and be out in nature. *We both liked to drink together as well, but let's leave that out for now.*

During one of my childhood moments where I'm sure I complained about something trivial, George set me straight based on his contrasting reality, which I had never experienced. George shared stories with me about growing up poor in a place called Atchison, Kansas, during the Dust Bowl, when nobody had any money. He later migrated to Omaha, met his wife-to-be, and they started out living on a floor of apartments that all shared one bathroom. His wife at that time was pregnant, just in case you thought that bathroom arrangement was bad enough. In the mornings he would go down to the job lines that were common during the Great Depression just to try to find work and make ends meet. George later worked for and then retired from the Railway Express Agency and Union Pacific Railroad shipping firearms across the country by train. Old pictures of him could easily be passed off for Indiana Jones. In these pictures he wore a fedora, leather jacket, and a pistol at his side. The similarities in looks alone between the two of them were simply uncanny!

George spent the majority of his life seeing parts of our country by train that most people will only read about in history books. He was also a master at guessing how many cars were connected to each passing train without even looking. It was not unusual to see him guess at train sizes during one of our hunting trips simply by listening to them pass way off in the distance. Every time we checked, he was almost always right—give or take a car or two. Now there's a talent I bet you've never heard of.

One of the greatest aspects of George was that despite the hardship of his earlier life, you would never hear him complain. That is, unless somebody didn't take American Express as a form of payment. He had an amazing outlook on life and even during the worst of times, he was always there to help anybody who needed him. He was a truly remarkable man and is still missed to this day. But just as George helped to "level-set" me at an earlier age, the lessons would keep coming later in my life as well, courtesy of my soon-to-be father-in-law, Tom.

I met Tom shortly after I started dating his daughter and my soon-to-be second-wife, Lisa, in New York. Lisa always spoke fondly of her father, and after meeting him I could understand why. Tom was always smiling and joking and had an amazing presence about him. *Why was this guy always so happy?* As I was soon to learn, Tom's contrast in life came at a very young age, during one of the darkest moments of the twentieth century.

Tom grew up as a young boy in Slovakia during the outbreak of World War II. When the Nazis invaded his country, Tom and his family were hidden in the attic of a house to elude the Nazis as they hunted down the Jews living in the area. During the latter half of the war, they were finally discovered and then shipped off to the Bergen-Belsen concentration camp in Germany, where they managed to survive for over six months until the end of the war and liberation by the British soldiers who first discovered the camp. Tom was six years old at the time of liberation and was lucky to be alive. Over fifty thousand people who were at that same camp were not as lucky, including the famous child diarist Anne Frank.

After the war his family was amazingly reunited on a train returning them to their home in Slovakia, where the Soviets were now in control and the persecution of the Jews continued. At that point they immigrated to the United States, taking what little the Soviets would let them escape with, and started a new life in the new world. Tom went on to become the youngest person to ever run a hospital system in New Jersey and, like many, despite his journey, was able to live out the American dream. Recently Tom revisited his childhood town and learned that a week after their capture from the attic where he and his family were hidden, an errant Allied bomb had dropped on that house and destroyed it. Had the Nazis not captured them when they did, he would surely be dead. *Fate plays us a very strange hand at times.* Tom will always be one of my heroes!

Speaking of fathers, people have asked me over the years what it was like losing my father at such a young age. Some even said they felt sorry for me, which I could never quite understand. People like George and later Tom taught me some of the most important lessons about life and, despite the pains of losing my father, I would hate to have lost these important times and lessons as well. Upon reflection, I also feel that our older population are perhaps our most under-utilized and under-appreciated people in our society today. I also wonder if it is any coincidence that as our generational gap increases so, too, does the suicide rate amongst those who could learn and benefit from them the most.

But despite losing my biological father, I did gain a wonderful stepfather only a few years later, which I will always be eternally thankful for. In many ways, Joe taught us many enduring life lessons that are still with me today. One of the most notable for me was taught during our first Christmas holiday seasons together in our new blended family. During that time, Joe asked us to join him in serving Christmas day breakfast to the homeless at the Siena/Francis House in downtown Omaha. Now, let me tell you, if you think your kids are spoiled and unappreciative, this is one of those life experiences that will help set them straight, and quickly!

There we all were, eagerly waiting Christmas day to arrive so we could finally open our presents under the tree that we had all guessed at a thousand times over. *Tie boxes were quickly ignored.* But just before we could receive our gifts, we had to first give to those who were truly much less fortunate than us. I will never forget how thankful and polite all the people we served were—it was both remarkable and eye-opening. Once we returned home, we couldn't help but feel a new sense of both appreciation and guilt for the gifts we were about to receive. Only hours before, people were thankful to us for simply being able to eat. Now, we were thankful for receiving even more action figures and ships to add to our ever-growing Star Wars collection. *It just didn't feel right anymore. Lesson learned.*

Now, with all the life lessons I have learned, I know you are probably waiting for my own profound answer to the question of why we are here, but I can only really answer that question for myself. Most people believe what they want to believe. I, however, know what I have experienced and touched on in this book, which leads me to a few undeniable conclusions of my own.

First, there is a higher being. You can call him what you want: God, Allah, Yahweh, Buddha, Shiva, Wakan Tanka, etc. I don't care. I know of some people during difficult times who have called him something different and even far worse but, despite all that, there was still a higher being. I personally grew up a Christian, so I guess I see God in a way that I can understand. Who knows? But that night when I was pulled into the light, heard a voice and commands, and experienced what I did, there was never a doubt in my mind that there was a God over all of us.

Second, we are a combination of body and spirit, which for some reason was designed that way for whatever God had planned for us. Our spirits (or souls) exist both before and after our bodies have died and I first realized this when I did not need my body for God to pull me away from it to give me my commands. This truth was further reaffirmed when a spirit decided, as previously discussed, to place itself within my physical body—presumably to send me a message or to seek some form of help.

Third, we are all here for a reason and a purpose, which we all seem to have to discover on our own. Whether you believe in them or not, commandments have been provided to man for thousands of years and I apparently received my own. I wish they were as easy to decipher as the Ten Commandments, but that was not my decision. The bottom line is, commandments or not, everybody is here for a reason and no matter what journey and destiny awaits us, it is all meant to be.

Finally, suicide is never an acceptable alternative or answer to life. Not in the eyes of those who love and care for you and not in the eyes of God. Those who knew David throughout his life like I did always knew that he was one of the nicest and most kind-hearted people they would ever meet. David always had a unique presence about him that people gravitated to whether he was truly aware of it or not. But David also struggled with life and society at times in a way that made him uneasy with the norms around him.

I remember us now-older kids were sitting in the waiting room at All Saints Episcopal Church *(Does this place finally sound familiar enough yet?)* prior to David's funeral service, when an attorney and close family friend named Russell ducked in for a quick moment as we all sat there staring at the floor in continued disbelief. I never forgot what Russell said to us that day. "David just didn't mechanically fit into this world." He went on to clarify that he wasn't referring to a true lack of mechanical reasoning that his father, Joe, suffered from when he scored in the lowest percentile in the nation as a child, causing his parents to take him in for tests to see if he was retarded *(their words, not mine)*. But we got the point the first time—David didn't always feel like he "fit in" to the world we live in, and anybody who knew David would never disagree with that summation.

David, like many other suicide victims I've read about, also had his bouts with substance abuse and depression throughout his life. It is unclear whether or not any of this "triggered" his final act of defiance, but I wouldn't rule it out, either. Despite the causes, for some reason David felt that suicide was a viable option for him, which to me is truly the greatest tragedy of all. By taking his own life, he also took from the lives of others at the same time. What may have seemed to him like an easy way to relieve his own pain caused it to be unknowingly transferred and amplified to others—namely those people he loved and who cared about him the most. Which always made me wonder: If the causing of harm to others in a mass shooting is so demented and wrong, then how is doing the same to those who care for you most while killing yourself any more acceptable? I realize this is a hard and uncomfortable question for many to ask but, to me, it is still worth asking.

Which brings me back to what we consider to be truly acceptable or unacceptable behavior in our lives. I recently read a press release published on the Journal of the American Academy of Child and Adolescent Psychiatry website comparing the suicide rates of teens both before and after the March 2017 release of Netflix's series *13 Reasons Why*, which featured the story of a seventeen-year-old boy who discovers cassette tapes outlining the thirteen reasons why his friend Hannah decided to end her life by suicide. According to the study, suicide rates increased by 28.9 percent for children ages ten to seventeen after the release of this series, which, at the time of this writing, was recently picked up for another season. Was this a coincidence? According to this study suicides dramatically spiked in the months immediately following the release of *13 Reasons Why*. To me that was a clear indication that it wasn't. So why are our youth so seemingly susceptible to suicide? And is this new?

For those of you who may be old enough to remember, a popular TV show called *M*A*S*H* ran from 1972 to 1983 and featured a group of Army surgeons based in South Korea during the Korean War. Each episode started with a very catchy song that, for those of you who remember, you can probably still hear playing in the back of your head even today. What you may not know, however, is the title of that song: "Suicide Is Painless."

As the story goes, the director of *M*A*S*H*, Robert Altman, had two stipulations for the new theme song for his show. First, it had to be called "Suicide Is Painless" and, second, it had to be "the stupidest song ever." After a failed attempt to write the lyrics himself, Altman assigned the task to his fourteen-year-old-son, who reportedly wrote the lyrics in only five minutes. *FIVE MINUTES!?* Let that sink in for a minute. A fourteen-year-old "child" was able to write the lyrics for a song about suicide being painless in five minutes only after a forty-five-year-old "man" could not. So, is it any coincidence, then, that ten-to-seventeen-year-olds have increased their suicide rates after the release of *13 Reasons Why?*

Unlike the lyrics to Altman's song, suicide is NOT painless. Yes, living life can be painful but, as my own experiences have shown me, that pain does not go away with suicide. It is simply transferred from one to others and, as my own experiences have taught me, can follow you into your next level of being as well. And who are the people in our world who may truly understand this the least? Our youth. To help clarify this point, just read the first three versus of the "stupidest song ever" to take a look into the mind of a fourteen-year-old:

> *Through early morning fog I see*
> *Visions of the things to be*
> *The pains that are withheld for me*
> *I realize and I can see*
> *That suicide is painless*
> *It brings on many changes*
> *And I can take or leave it if I please*
> *The game of life is hard to play*
> *I'm gonna lose it anyway*
> *The losing card I'll someday lay*
> *So this is all I have to say*

So, as you can see, the only pain released by suicide is the pain that lives on with others, making suicide truly the most selfish act anyone could ever carry out. Yet in the case of David, it came from one of the most unselfish and caring people I have ever known. I still believe in my heart that David would never knowingly want to pass on so much pain and misery to those who loved him, which is why I believe that we need to create greater awareness of the true impacts of suicide on people if we are ever going to stop this from happening again.

Speaking of happening again, I, like many of you, have been part of discussions where somebody has asked, "If you could go back in history and spend a day with anybody, who would it be?" After August 25, 2002, this was always an easy answer for me. I would trade nearly anything for one chance to go back in time to try to save the life of my brother David. But as my own experiences have shown me, at least God gave me a chance to help try to save his soul instead.

Shortly after my many countless prayers and demands of David to look beyond the grey sky and to seek out and follow the light, everything eventually stopped. No more gut-punching visits, no more aimless experiences at night lost in the woods with David, and no more questions in my mind as to where my brother is today.

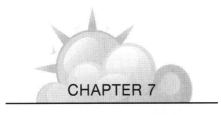

CHAPTER 7

FINDING HOPE

"Only in the darkness can you see the stars."

—Dr. Martin Luther King Jr.

"Hope is being able to see that there is light despite all the darkness."

—Desmond Tutu

Louis Zamperini was a remarkable man who lived an amazing life story. After running for the US in the Berlin Olympics in 1936, he later served on a B-24 bomber in the Pacific in World War II. While conducting a search mission over the Pacific, his bomber crashed into the ocean, killing eight of the eleven crew members. For the next forty-seven days, Louis and the two other surviving crew members were set adrift with no food or water on a small life raft never designed for such endurance.

On day thirty-three, one of the crew members, Francis McNamara, gave up hope and died, leaving Louis and Russell Allen Phillips as the only two remaining survivors when they finally reached land in the Japanese-controlled Marshall Islands.

But that was only the beginning of Louis's life trials as he would continue to endure seemingly endless torture and abuse at the hands of his Japanese captors until the end of the war. His story of survival and ability to endure unspeakable abuse as a prisoner of war was so inspiring that it later became a bestselling book and Hollywood movie entitled Unbroken. In reflecting on his life journey, Louis once stated, "To persevere, I think, is important for everybody. Don't give up, don't give in. There's always an answer to everything."

Stories of survival and incredible human perseverance can be seen throughout history and are frequently told in times of war. What makes each story so compelling is how some people will endure almost any level of pain and suffering when so many others will not. People gravitate to such stories because the people we tend to admire most are the ones who overcame so much adversity in their lives. Shakespeare understood this better than anyone when he created stories based on "the hero's journey," a format that is still used today in many of our most admired books and movies. *So, what is it that compels certain people to persevere through extreme levels of pain and suffering while others will more quickly succumb to a more tragic fate and even give up on life?*

In this chapter, I will share my personal observations, reflections, and recommendations to help answer this question based on my own life experiences, many of which I have discussed in this book. I do this fully realizing that others may disagree or have different conclusions based on their own experiences, religious teachings, and beliefs. It is not my intent to disagree with any other viewpoints on this matter but rather to share my own observations and beliefs to help broaden everyone's observations on this topic. For if my own observations can help save at least one additional life from suicide, then it will be worth the effort to me.

As previously discussed, my own experiences have shown me that as humans, we live our lives as two entities operating as one. Our body is the form we were given to best survive in this world and our soul lives within our bodies. I start here because this lack of fundamental understanding of our very existence is what, in my opinion, continues to fail so many people. For what is needed to survive and grow in our physical existence is not what is needed to grow in our spiritual existence as well—both need to grow up and mature in their own ways.

Our bodies require food, water, and oxygen to survive and grow. This is the form we have taken, and this is what is required to grow and maintain it. But if our bodily survival alone were enough, why do some people like Louis Zamperini survive through extreme levels of bodily pain and suffering when others do not? To me, it is because the human soul also requires something that compels it to survive and grow. That something is called hope.

Hope is the sustainable lifeforce of the soul. Hope allows us to endure pain, hardship, and suffering. Hope allows us to sacrifice so we and the others who follow us don't have to. Hope wills us to want better in our lives and the lives of those we care for. Hope allows us to take risks to help us improve life. Hope allows for acceptance. And most importantly, hope allows us to want to grow, for we are all here for a reason and as such, we can better grow and do more good for others by living life through challenges and overcoming obstacles in our own ways.

In my own life, hope has allowed me to endure my own pains and suffering and has taught me that through these trials and tribulations, I am a stronger and wiser person as a result. Losing my brother to suicide was perhaps the most painful trial of my life but through hope, I can now find meaning from it. Suicide is a national and worldwide epidemic and as long as it continues, I know that what I have experienced can now help me share my story with others and hopefully help to save future lives. Suicide is not the answer and we all need to better understand that there is hope for every life in this world despite all of the suffering and pain each and every one of us endures as humans.

In order to find hope in my own life, I, like so many other people, have struggled at times with my own journey to understanding until I was able to better organize and manage it into the three most critical elements I refer to as **the three P's: PRESENCE, PASSION, and PURPOSE**. Here is how to understand each in more detail.

The first is our ability to better understand and manage our own **PRESENCE**. I truly believe that even though all people are influenced by their cultures and surroundings, in the end all people are self-determining and therefore responsible for making their own choices in life. And one of the greatest choices we can make is defining our own presence. When it comes to managing our presence, I break this down into three areas: knowing WHERE you stand in the world, HOW you stand, and WHO you stand with.

Your **WHERE** starts with understanding where your "happy place" is in the world and then pursuing it. If you ever watched the movie *Happy Gilmore*, you will remember Happy visualizing his happy place, which allowed him to better focus and pursue his goals. As comedic and crazy as this movie was, there was a lot of value in this one point, and you need to do the same thing. Start by closing your eyes and seeing yourself in your own happy place. Once you see it, now you need to pursue it. What are you doing? Who are you with? And perhaps most importantly, where are you located? In America, you always have forty-nine other choices, so if your happy place is not where you are now, move. How do you think a Nebraska boy like me ended up in Arizona? Arizona was my happy place and now I am living the dream and you should be, too.

Speaking of moving, I have always believed that in the United States, there is a state that best matches each person's personality. Even though I grew up in Nebraska, I love the outdoors and hate cold weather. So, when I was old enough, I chose to change my presence and eventually made it to Arizona. What amazes me is how many people won't do the same thing. Most people in the world are stuck where they live and many can never move to improve their presence in life. But Americans are incredibly lucky and can simply hop in a car and radically change their *where* for the better in a matter of hours. That is, unless something is holding them back.

A growing concern I have for both America and the world is the growing level of debt being incurred by our younger generations. In America alone, student debt has now reached $1.5 trillion! To put this into perspective, if our student debt alone were its own economy, it would rank near the twelfth largest in the world—on par with Canada and Russia. High levels of debt in a free market economy can stifle mobility within the workforce and tie people into living and working conditions that can seem inescapable. Carrying such high levels of personal debt can also create a lot of stress and anxiety and is frequently mentioned as the primary cause for younger adults who claim to have no meaning or purpose in their lives. For this reason alone, I highly recommend that people find ways to control and eliminate high levels of personal debt—especially incurred by our youngest generations. Nobody should have to start their adult lives by first digging themselves out of a deep hole that can take years or even decades to remove themselves from.

The second area of your presence is **HOW** you present yourself to others. When people meet you and get to know you, do they like you? Do they respect you? Or do they dislike you? Be honest when asking these questions of yourself. The most important aspect of how you control the *how* of your presence is ironically 100 percent always in your control. We call this your attitude. Nothing can change the *how* of your presence faster and better than a change in your attitude. You will notice it and others will notice it as well, and just like good karma, how you treat others will come back to you.

One of the best ways to start improving your attitude is to remove as much negativity as possible from your presence. For most people, this can start with what you chose to see and hear on a daily basis. I remember a conversation I had many years ago with the former mayor of Omaha, who lost his son to suicide. He told me that kids need to stop watching the news because it is so negative. Since that time, cable news has grown to providing us with a perpetual twenty-four-hour news cycle that is filled with negativity. It's little wonder to me that the rapid decline in the political discourse in our country happened at the same time as the emergence of the twenty-four-hour news cycle. If you are still not convinced, turn on any of the major cable news channels for three hours and ask yourself how you feel after watching it.

An equally important aspect of attitude simply comes from controlling your own thoughts. What you think ultimately manifests itself into who you are and what you become. If you think negatively of the world and the people around you and in your life, that is what you will project to others. The opposite is also true. That is why it is so important to block and remove negative thoughts from your life; it's one of the greatest ways you can control negativity at the source.

Another important consideration of your *how* comes from how you dress. People often forget that the first statement you make to others happens the minute you walk through the door—before you ever say a word! This is why you should always dress for the life you want and not the life you have. Just like with your attitude, how you dress is a self-fulfilling prophecy to the life you ultimately want to live and even though some people today might disagree with this suggestion, they are also likely to be the ones who never aspire to improve the *how* of their own presence. So always consider the source of any criticism.

The third aspect of your presence is better managing **WHO** you are present with in this world. I am sure you have heard the old saying that if you show me your friends, I'll show you your future. This is absolutely true and when it comes to people, birds of a feather will flock together, so make sure the people you decide to befriend, network with, work with, and love are people who share the same life goals and values that you aspire to. This applies just as much to your work life as it does your personal life.

For example, after I sold my last software company, I received a phone call from a former employee of mine named Andrew. Andrew had been working for a new digital marketing company and thought I should join them. What I didn't know at the time was I would end up working for this new company for over a decade, which is almost unheard of in our industry. But the glue that really made this organization so unique were 130 of the absolute best salespeople in the industry, who developed such a strong and unique culture that we referred to each other as "family." Many of these people who moved on over the years often brought other work family members with them to even better opportunities— without them even applying for another job. Hell, I'm pretty sure most of these people didn't even have a résumé ready, and probably never would need one again. Birds of a feather . . .

Once you start taking the steps to improve your presence in life, you will be doing what many great people before you have done as well. Throughout history, we know that most great people have improved their presence to find meaning and success in their lives. So can you. When you reflect on these changes, you will also better understand that what we see and know is greatly impacted by what we experience and learn. This is referred to as "the contrast principle" and, as previously discussed, helps to govern so many decisions we make each day in our lives, including how we look at money.

One of the biggest misconceptions we have is that somehow money can buy us happiness. If we only had more money our problems would somehow go away. Right? Wrong! Money doesn't solve problems, it only creates new ones; there is no amount of money that can solve the problems that we create with and without it. This is why there are so many stories of famous athletes and lottery winners who started with nothing, suddenly became flush with money, and then ended up losing it all in the end. That is also why it is so important to start working on improving your presence in your own life, which will help you with the second "P": PASSION.

Nothing great in life is ever accomplished without **PASSION**. Passion is what allows ordinary people to accomplish extraordinary things. Passion is what burns deep inside each and every one of us when we are at our best doing what we can do best. The problem with passion, however, is that far too many people live and work without it and don't even realize it until it's too late. Some even struggle to understand what they are truly passionate about to begin with. When I hear these comments from others, I commonly ask, "Have you ever done something in your life that you were so passionate about that once you looked up at the clock you asked yourself where all the time went?" Ask yourself this same question and start writing those instances down, for over time, as I have witnessed in my own life, many of your passions can evolve and change.

When it comes to passion, it is important to remember that all of us are born with various God-given talents and no two people are the same. Passion will likely be different for everybody. The most important thing to remember is to always seek out and find passion at every stage in your life. Your passions may and likely will change over time, but your need for passion will not. That is why when some passions leave you, you need to let go and find new passions to replace them. Sadly, we sometimes see this need in full effect when we hear stories about older couples who are passionately married for countless years and when one spouse dies, the other quickly follows. Many will then comment that the second spouse died of "a broken heart." What they are really saying is that they lost their passion in life and didn't replace it. This same pattern is also commonly witnessed with successful businesspeople who, once they retire, tend to lose the one passion— work—that governed so much of their lives. It is not uncommon to hear how these people seem to "quickly age" once their work life is past them—and who wants to retire so you can age quicker?

Looking back at my own childhood, I led a rather unorthodox life and was frequently referred to as a black sheep by many who knew me. At the age of fifteen, I built and raced my first NASCAR race car when many of my friends did otherwise—or in some cases did nothing at all. It was a highly expensive and time-consuming process that took up nearly all of my free time in my teens. I became so passionate about building and racing stock cars that in many ways it consumed my life at that time with hard work, joy, and fulfillment. It was only after I left for college and stopped racing that I realized I had lost my passion with nothing to replace it with.

Like many college freshmen, I was simply not ready for nor passionate about my college studies. I remember pulling out a large stack of pictures of my old race cars and staring aimlessly at them for hours on end, trying to get my passion back while studying a major in college that was flat-out boring to me. I was literally living without passion that year and my grades clearly reflected it—I damn near flunked out. It was only when I took a new course entitled Personal Finance 201 my sophomore year that a light went on in me and I rediscovered my passion again and ended up graduating on the Dean's List of the Business College.

Over the course of my life, my passions have changed and evolved but I always knew that I could never live without passion ever again. When one passion would lapse or lose its significance it was always my goal to find another one to replace it. For a life lived with passion is the difference between living and existing, and our souls were not placed here merely to exist. Which takes us to the third of my "P's," which will help you fuel your passions. That is PURPOSE.

So, what is the **PURPOSE** of life and how do you find it? This has been a burning question that the human race has been asking ourselves since the dawn of our existence and I'm not sure we are getting any closer to an answer—especially amongst our youth. I recently ran across a 2019 poll conducted by Yakult UK, which found that 89 percent of Gen-Zers (ages 18–29) felt their life was meaningless and had no purpose. This number dropped to 80 percent for respondents of all ages and 55 percent for people over the age of 60.[1] In summary, the majority of people in the UK, and the vast majority of their youth, are living lives without meaning and purpose. So, what does this really mean? And was Benjamin Franklin correct when

1 Sun Reporter, 2019. "Millennial Melancholy: Nine in ten young Brits believe their life lacks purpose, according to shocking new study." The Sun. https://www.thesun.co.uk/news/9637619/young-brits-life-lacks-purpose/ (accessed September 23, 2019)

he said "Many people die at twenty-five and aren't buried until they are seventy-five?"

Famed psychologist and Holocaust survivor Viktor E. Frankl argued that life is primarily a quest for meaning. This theory contrasted with other leading thinkers in his profession, who argued that life is a quest for pleasure (as Sigmund Freud believed), or a quest for power (as Alfred Adler believed). In man's ultimate search for meaning, Frankl argued that people are more tempted to distract themselves with pleasure when meaning is absent in their lives. Frankl pointed to research indicating a strong relationship with "meaningless" and addictions, criminal behaviors, and depression. Therefore, without meaning, people fill this void with hedonistic pleasures, materialism, quests for power, drug use, hatred, compulsions, and boredom.

Frankl also witnessed a direct connection between a lack of meaning in life and suicide. In the 1930s, Frankl spent four years at Austria's largest state hospital treating more than twelve thousand patients—most of whom had previously attempted suicide. Most of his patients had told him afterward that they were now happy that their attempts to kill themselves had failed. In the weeks, months, and years that followed their attempts, most told him upon reflection that there actually had been a solution to their problem and a meaning to their lives.[2]

---

2 Viktor E. Frankl, 2006, Man's Search For Meaning (Boston: Beacon Press), 142.

Frankl used this experience throughout his life to tell others in similar situations why they too had to live to see the day when they would find these answers to their own life as well. His contention was that for most, the final meaning of life may not fully reveal itself until the end of our lives. Therefore, the greatest pursuit in any life is to find meaning by living out our entire lives, for meaning and purpose are what compels us to survive and grow through all of life's obstacles. Or as Nietzsche famously said, "He who has a WHY to live for can bear almost any HOW." This means a determination of living through all stages of life as well.

Shakespeare said that every person goes through seven stages of life, ranging from infancy to our imminent death. By studying Shakespeare and each one of these stages, we realize that meaning and purpose can change and evolve as your life changes, which is why it is important to never give up on your life journey by intentionally cutting it short. No matter how much pain and suffering you may have to endure through any one of these stages, it is necessary for your soul to journey through all of these experiences and help fulfill God's purpose for you in the world—which you will then carry with you into the next. By intentionally cutting this journey short through suicide, you are making a choice to cut short this important spiritual journey that was planned for you to help your soul become stronger for what lies ahead after you die.

Remember, we are all here for a reason and for a purpose—whether you know it yet or not. Some may know their meaning and purpose the day they are born while many may only discover it upon their death. Mark Twain was famous for saying, "The two most important days in your life are the day you are born and the day you find out why." The objective is to never give up and always try to find purpose and meaning in everything that happens in your life, through both the good and the bad.

In my own life, as previously explained, I received my calling in my late twenties. Apparently, somebody upstairs wasn't happy with how I was handling my life up to that point, leading to me getting called out on it. In this one brief but life-altering experience, I was given a message that I did not truly comprehend until years later, when I was able to find a way to turn a tragedy into meaning and purpose in my own life—which ultimately led to this book and telling this story to the world. But not everybody may receive, nor will they need, their own calling to help discover their own meaning and purpose in life. There are ways we can try to discover this on our own.

To help answer the question of how to discover your purpose in life, I have reflected on six key questions that have helped me determine this answer for myself. These include:

WHAT ARE YOUR GOD-GIVEN TALENTS?
When I received my calling, I was clearly getting the message that I was dropping the ball on the talent front. When I was told to stop wasting my talents, naturally the first question I had for myself was "What exactly are my talents?" I had never really contemplated this question up to this point because my life had been motivated largely based on the passions and ambitions of a younger aspiring businessman. I began to ask myself these questions over and over again but only when I began asking these questions of others did the picture start becoming clearer to me.

Self-reflection is a powerful tool in life, but to self-critique can be far more difficult when looking through our own distorted lenses of ourselves. That is why it is always a good idea to start by asking others you know what talents they see in you that perhaps you don't see in yourself. Then ask them what they think you were really meant to do in life. You might be surprised by the answers you receive—I was. One example in my own life started to come into focus after I did exactly this.

In my life and work, I do a lot of writing and public speaking. I have been told by many people who have heard me speak that I was "born to be a speaker." But what they don't know was I was not always able to speak this well, and that only after I was able to learn and master public speaking did it become a powerful tool in my life. But the indications that I could and should do public speaking well were there long before I really knew it and only through reflection was I able to truly see it. One such example came from my confirmation at church.

At that time, I was asked along with another member of my class to speak to our congregation. Normally, people don't come naturally to public speaking—especially as young children. In fact, it is commonly known that people are more fearful of public speaking than dying, so clearly it is not preferred by most. But when I thought back to this speech later in life, one of the things that struck me was how I felt when I delivered it. I had no fear whatsoever when speaking in front of a large congregation. In fact, not only was there no fear, but there was also a heightened level of clarity, energy, thinking, and even joy in what I was doing—all of which are still with me today. The signs were clearly there at a young age but only when I worked to develop the mechanics of speaking did I realize that this was truly something I was meant to do.

Once you start reflecting on your own talents and asking others for help, start making a list of all of your talents while placing the most obvious ones at the top of your list.

WHAT ARE YOU PASSIONATE ABOUT NOW? What do you really love to do more than anything else? What tends to come easy for you? By understanding what you love and what comes easy for you you can quickly separate your potentially aspirational and unrealistic dreams from your God-given reality. After all, we are not all cut out to be movie stars and professional athletes, now, are we? Remember, everyone is unique and is born with unique talents and it is your job to discover what yours are, starting now. If you get stuck here, ask yourself what you love to do now—the things that make you feel like time runs out and you forget to eat, sleep, or go to the bathroom when you do them. These are indications of your current passions. Start making a list of these things in order of your level of passion for them.

WHAT MOMENTS/EVENTS HAVE MADE YOU HAPPIEST IN YOUR LIFE? What things have brought the greatest joy to you? What moments stand out in your life as the greatest moments and when you seemed happiest? Again, make a list with the happiest moments at the top.

IF YOU KNEW YOU HAD ONLY ONE MORE YEAR TO LIVE, HOW WOULD YOU CHANGE YOUR LIFE NOW TO SPEND THESE LAST 365 DAYS ON EARTH? There are many stories of people who escaped sudden death and changed their lives forever as a result. In the face of death, some made promises to God while others made promises to themselves that if they could only live longer, they would change their life for the better. What fundamentally changed for nearly all of these people was the sudden and real feeling of transience they now felt in their life knowing that it could all suddenly end in an instant. For other people in similar realities, the end came much slower, but the feelings and observations were very similar.

Steve Jobs was arguably one of the most innovative and impactful business leaders of our time. In the year leading up to his death in 2011, Jobs took a leave of absence and later resigned from his position as CEO of Apple to help fight what ultimately became a terminal bout with cancer. During that time, Jobs famously stated upon contemplating his own imminent death: "Remembering that I'll be dead soon is the most important tool I've ever encountered to help me make the big choices in life. Almost everything—all external expectations, all pride, all fear of embarrassment or failure—these things just fall away in the face of death, leaving only what is truly important. Remembering that you are going to die is the best way I know to avoid the trap of thinking you have something to lose. You are already naked. There is no reason not to follow your heart."

What Jobs so eloquently illustrated in his remarks is not dissimilar to how many people reflect on their lives in the end. But sadly, too many people face the end of their lives with far too many regrets about how they should have lived their lives in the first place. In 2009, an Australian palliative care nurse named Bronnie Ware wrote an article on her blog titled *Regrets of the Dying*, in which she summarized the top five regrets of her patients who were living through and reflecting on the last twelve weeks of their lives.[3] These regrets included . . .

I wish I'd had the courage to live a life true to myself, not the life others expected of me. Most people Bronnie interviewed indicated that they had not honored even half of their dreams and had to die knowing that this was the result of choices they had made or not made in their own lives.

I wish I hadn't worked so hard. This feedback came from every male patient she nursed in their final days. Many had indicated that they'd missed their children's youth and their partner's companionship—all sacrificed for their work.

I wish I'd had the courage to express my feelings. Many people indicated that they suppressed their feelings in order to keep peace with others in their lives. As a result, they settled for

3 Bronnie Ware, 2019. "Regrets of the Dying." BronnieWare. com Blog. https://bronnieware.com/blog/regrets-of-the-dying/ (accessed August 22, 2019)

a mediocre existence and never became who they were truly capable of becoming. Many developed illnesses related to the bitterness and resentment they carried as a result.

I wish I had stayed in touch with my friends. There were many deep regrets about not giving friendships the time and effort they deserved. Everyone indicated that they missed their friends when they were dying.

I wish that I had let myself be happier. Bronnie indicated that many did not realize until the end that *happiness is a choice.* They had stayed stuck in old patterns and habits. The so-called "comfort" of familiarity overflowed into their emotions as well as their physical lives. Fear of change had them pretending to others, and to themselves, that they were content, when deep within they longed to laugh properly and have silliness in their lives again.

So ask yourself the question about the end of your life once again and write down your answers with the most important changes you would make first. Start reflecting: Is there anywhere on your list where you indicated that you wanted to give up on your dreams, work harder, not express your true feelings, become a worse friend, and let yourself be more miserable in life? Now ask yourself how long it will take for you to finally realize this before it is too late and you end up repeating the same life regrets shared by Bronnie's patients.

WHAT HAVE YOU LEARNED FROM YOUR MISTAKES AND BAD EXPERIENCES IN LIFE? As humans, we can only learn through reflection, and EVERYBODY deals with suffering, pain, struggles, and problems through our spiritual journey through life—both rich and poor. And once again, don't think that money alone will solve your problems, for it will not. Money doesn't solve problems—it only creates new ones. So, begin by asking yourself: How have your most difficult experiences helped you grow stronger as a person? What meaning and purpose have you found for each and every one of them? Remember, some of our greatest spiritual growth often comes from our greatest struggles in life. Or as Nietzsche said, "That which does not kill us makes us stronger." You also don't have to learn from only your own struggles; many lessons can be learned from the struggles of others as well. So start by making a list of your biggest mistakes and worst experiences in your life and then indicate what you have learned from each and every one of them.

FINALLY, WHAT WOULD PEOPLE MISS ABOUT YOU (PERSONALLY AND PROFESSIONALLY) IF YOU WERE NO LONGER HERE? In 1946, one the greatest holiday classic movies of all time, *It's a Wonderful Life*, was released in theaters. Since its release, it is not uncommon to see regular reruns of this classic movie on TV during the holiday seasons. In this movie, George Bailey, played by Jimmy Stewart, tries to take his own life only to be saved by an angel who shows him what his town and family would look like without him. It was this stark contrast of reality that shocked George into realizing just how important his life was to everybody around him and why ending his life would be such a tragedy in so many ways.

Fortunately for George Bailey, he was given a second chance, but for people who end up taking their own lives, this second chance will never come. That is why it is so important for everybody to truly consider and reflect on what people would miss most about you if you were gone. What impact would it have on your family members, friends, and those who love you? What would be the impact on your community, work environment, and contributions to society? Start making a list of all the negative potential impacts this could cause. If you struggle with this question, start by asking the people closest to you this same question and see what they say.

By asking these six questions of yourself and reviewing them frequently, you can help to both understand yourself better and discover how to find your own meaning, purpose, and hope in life. I would also encourage you to not compare the journey of your life to others, for I believe that God created everybody with their own unique talents and purposes and therefore some may not always fit the mold of what others might consider to be the societal norm—which is fine. In the case of my brother David, I believe that his inherent conflict between who he truly was deep down and what others expected of him led to a great deal of pain and suffering in his own heart and mind. In my opinion, my brother could have learned a great deal by asking these six questions of himself but, sadly, unlike George Bailey, he never gave himself a second chance to try to find the hope, meaning, and purpose in his own life that may have helped to save him. And as we continue to witness with tragic consequences, the loss of hope in one's life can have deadly consequences.

So, one of the greatest lessons I have learned in my life is that hope truly is the sustainable lifeforce of the soul, and even when we have enough to live with, without hope, we can have nothing to live for. What feeds our bodily growth cannot feed the growth of our soul and our spiritual journey throughout our lives. Only hope can provide this fuel, and through improvements in our own presence, passions, and purpose we can help provide meaning and hope so we can all continue our spiritual journeys as planned. It is therefore my opinion that only when all of us—people of all races, religions, cultures, and even those who are consumed by nihilism—can come to this realization will the epidemic of suicides in our country and worldwide decline and change for the better.

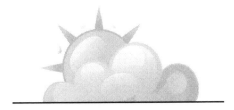

EPILOGUE

It has been seventeen years since the day David took his own life. Since then time has marched on and, in the words of my mother, time has worked on healing old wounds. With each passing month and year, the shock and disbelief of David's death becomes a little less painful but never fully goes away. I often compare the passing of time after a suicide to how nuclear scientists view the storage of nuclear waste.

For scientists, radioactive isotopes eventually decay and disintegrate, commonly measured in "half-lives." Accordingly, each half-life represents half the loss of power and the danger that goes with it. Even though it will not fully go away, it can reach tolerable and even livable levels. The point being, the harm and dangers will dissipate over time but they never fully go away. The same is true for the pain felt by the survivors of suicide. It never fully disappears and, like nuclear waste, burying it deep inside a mountain (or your mind) to decay doesn't make it simply "go away." But as hard as this reality has become, my family has "survived" and moved on the best they can.

Our oldest brother, Scott, has become the Right Reverend J Scott Barker—Bishop of Nebraska's Episcopal Diocese. We all loved seeing Scott return home but nobody was prouder the day Scott moved back to become Bishop of Nebraska than his father, Joe. A lot of special traditions exist in families, but to have one that spans over one hundred years in the same location is quite remarkable and is what some would even call fate. I once asked Scott why he quit law school to begin divinity school and his journey into the priesthood, and he said it was simple: He got his calling. *Clearly Scott's calling was much less of a riddle than mine.*

My sister, Amy, currently resides in Memphis, Tennessee, with her husband and two children, for as long as Cliff stays at FedEx, I suppose. My relationship with Amy didn't start out on the right foot when our family first formed but as the years progressed, I have grown to love her like a sister. Amy inherited her father's charming personality and work ethic, which have shown brightly throughout her life. Amy's personality is magnetic and I have commonly joked over the years that if you placed her in Antarctica for a year she would eventually befriend every penguin around.

Doug is currently an attorney in private practice in Omaha and is married with two children. Like the rest of us, Doug has become more "tame" over time and now longs for, amongst other things, the perfect outcome of four hours on grass, which most people refer to as golf. As much as I love golf, I also understand the definition of insanity, which is why I love our "occasional" family golf outings versus Doug's multi-weekly ritual of inspecting his last divots at Champions Run. When people commonly refer to somebody's spouse as being their "better half," they often say it in jest. In Doug's case, his wife, Laurie, has truly made him a better man and father and is well deserving of that title. *Most of our wives are, for the matter.*

David's father, Joe, died a little over three years ago now, and I asked, as I always try to do to help honor those closest to me who have impacted my life, to speak at his funeral. I wanted to make Joe's eulogy a short story of his life, full of wonderful stories and lessons we have learned from him. Of course, the summary of his life journey would not have been complete had I not mentioned the loss of his son David and the impact it had on his life. As previously mentioned, public speaking comes unusually naturally for me, but this was the part of his eulogy I struggled to get through. I even stopped at this point to apologize to those in attendance while I tried to fight back my own emotions that were choking me up.

Joe was like most people—he had both his wonderful qualities and some vices. *We are all human.* Fortunately, his vices were little, self-inflicted, and were often devoid of any of the logic I had once learned in Statistics 101. Joe was a great and loving father and stepfather, with few regrets. As previously mentioned, Joe loved to sing and he once told me that his biggest regret in life was not making the Yale Whiffenpoofs singing group during his time at Yale. Much like a jigsaw puzzle that is missing a piece, Joe and I were inherently very different people. But that didn't mean I didn't love him. It just took me time to better understand and appreciate him for who he was. But throughout all that, Joe was always there for me when I needed him the most and, in the end, that is all that really mattered to me.

Our mother DEDE is doing what DEDE does best—she is living life to the fullest. It is hard to describe how remarkable a person my mother truly is. Perhaps the best way to sum up her impact on other people comes from when I run into old friends who are years and even decades removed from the old days in Omaha. And who do they ask about first? You guessed it . . . DEDE. Many words could be used to describe Mom: a survivor, friendly, gregarious, charming, beautiful, caring, strong, resilient, and the list goes on. Of course, I am biased! *Who the hell isn't when describing their own mother?* But for the people who know her best, I am confident that all would agree with my description.

DEDE has now been widowed twice over and helped raise five children into this world. She and Joe beat remarkable odds in raising a highly diverse blended family with all of the trials and tribulations that come with it. *Which were many, thanks to us little shits.* Much like her father, George, before her, DEDE continues to remain the life of any party and one of the greatest role models I know for what life is really all about. In the end, Mom has lived, experienced, and accomplished more in one lifetime than most of us could ever imagine, and in doing so she has always persevered with elegance and charm. *What a great role model.*

David's wife, Amy, has since remarried and still resides in Omaha raising two beautiful children. Amy and I were in the same grade growing up and frequented many of the same social circles during that time. She was always very kind and had a crush on David for as long as I could remember when we were growing up. They eventually tied the knot in a beautiful wedding in her parents' backyard and lived together for the last years of David's life. Since David's death, Amy's and my worlds have grown apart. As much as I wanted to better stay in touch, I also wanted her to move on with her life without any further painful memories that my own experiences could have brought to her. She of all people deserves to be happy again and I just couldn't look her straight in the face without knowing in the back of my mind what was happening. None of this was her fault, yet I'm sure her pain was greater than anybody's as a result. *I still feel terrible for Amy.*

As for myself, well, life has never been dull. My first marriage lasted seven years and even though we could not make it work, we have two wonderful children as a result. I had a divorce attorney once tell me that marriage is like making pancakes—you always throw out the first one. So, I guess that is what we did. *Good advice – but always try to avoid it if you can!* I have since found love again and after a number of years living in New York, Lisa and I decided to chase my childhood dream of living somewhere closer to my personality and now are happily married and reside in Arizona. I have always believed that each person has a state that best matches their personality and character, and I knew at a young age that Arizona was the closest state to mine. Nebraska by birth, Arizona by choice. Despite my choice, I am still and will always be a rabid Huskers fan, which is something that my son, Chase—despite never having lived in Nebraska—now shares with me.

Like most people, my life continues to be filled with more questions than answers. The riddle of my calling still haunts me to this day. What are my talents and am I still wasting them? After all, nobody wants to reach the pearly gates one day only to have the Big Man greet you with "Didn't you get my message?" As for my talents, I do a lot of public speaking and writing in my work and both seem to come unusually naturally to me. I have been told by a number of people I have worked with over the years that this is my gift. But are these also my talents? Perhaps—time will tell. I guess as long as I wasn't destined to become a rodeo clown, I should be okay.

As for David, I believe he has finally reached a place where life in this world and the next make more sense to him now. When he was alive, David would advise others to "follow their bliss," which, in hindsight, may have been much more a struggle for David to do for himself than anybody really knew until it was too late. During David's life he lived through both the common and countercultures of our society. He tried new experiences, followed his heart, and always remained true to himself and others. He loved and gave willingly and graciously to all and especially to those who were close to him, and he frequently asked for little or nothing in return. He was a beautiful person who had his own compass in life. But in the end, that was apparently not enough. Instead, the answers that seemed to elude him have now become questions and pains that we all, as survivors of suicide, must learn to live with.

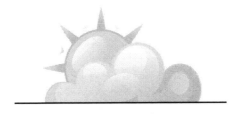

LIKE THIS BOOK?

If so, please provide a review
and order additional copies today at:

BeyondTheGreySky.com

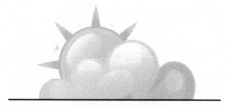

NOTES

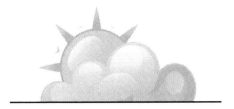

NOTES

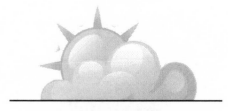

NOTES

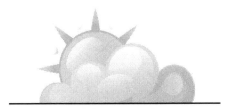

NOTES

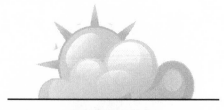

NOTES

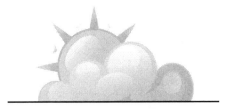

NOTES

Made in the USA
San Bernardino, CA
21 May 2020

72052285R00095